DIARY OF A
RADICAL CANCER WARRIOR

*To HCC
Students

With love*

DIARY OF A
RADICAL CANCER WARRIOR

FIGHTING CANCER AND CAPITALISM
AT THE CELLULAR LEVEL

FRED HO

FOREWORD BY MAGDALENA GÓMEZ
INTRODUCTION BY CYNTHIA G. FRANKLIN

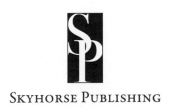

Skyhorse Publishing

Skyhorse Publishing books may be purchased in bulk at special discounts for sales promotion, corporate gifts, fund-raising, or educational purposes. Special editions can also be created to specifications. For details, contactthe Special Sales Department, Skyhorse Publishing, 307 West 36th Street, 11th Floor, New York, NY 10018 or info@skyhorsepublishing.com.

Skyhorse® and Skyhorse Publishing® are registered trademarks of Skyhorse Publishing, Inc.®, a Delaware corporation.

www.skyhorsepublishing.com

10 9 8 7 6 5 4 3 2 1

Library of Congress Cataloging-in-Publication Data available on file.
ISBN: 978-1-61608-378-6

Printed in the United States of America

All love to my original Warriors for Fred/Circle of Love/ *kokuas*: Ann T. Greene, Magdalena Gómez, Paget Walker, and Jennifer Feil.

To all the *kokuas* (many of whom are named in this book), my family, to my medical team (Drs. Richard Emmanuel, Evan Berman, Dilip Patel, Antonio Picon, Peter Kozuch, Chip Foley, Sovrin Shah, Kenneth Hu, Bill Akpinar and his staff, Umi, Amy, Carlos, Danny, Brittney, Francoisse, Barney, Fran, Charlene Muhmmad, Joseph Harris, Chao Chen), and all nurses and staff at all the hospitals and medical centers that saw me through this brutal war and incredible journey of transformation.

To Cynthia Franklin for immediately agreeing to write the wonderful introduction and to Magdalena for writing the very moving foreword.

To Paul Lyons, fellow radical cancer warrior, who made the introduction to Skyhorse Publishing.

CONTENTS

PART TWO:

The War Returns—Rejecting the Allopathic for the Naturopathic

Foreword

Fred Ho's cancer diaries are a life-affirming journey of one person's struggle in the fight for his life. Fred's diaries encourage not only the cancer patient but also friends, family, and colleagues whose lives are also affected by the shock and unfolding of this insidious modern-day disease.

The voice of these diaries is reflective, philosophical, inquisitive, humorous, challenging, political, and blunt—one that never succumbs to the most understandable temptation of self-pity. It is all too common to feel alone, not only as the patient but also as a care provider; at some point in the day the backwash of helplessness slaps us down. These diaries are an antidote to feelings of despair, victimization, and surrender. Fred is not a victim of cancer, but its formidable opponent.

Fred takes us on his daily excursions of treatment, symptoms, self-advocacy, and care. His authentic, provocative voice provides the reader with viable, practical tools to take charge when facing cancer or any enemy that would attempt to subjugate the quality of one's life. Through the simplicity of honest reflection, Fred brings patient and care providers out of isolation. Look up his recipe for rehydration, or his rediscovery of the healing properties of house plants. Walk with him and find joy in the simple moments of life: tasting a fresh basil leaf, biting into a steamed pork bun, breathing deeply through the Brooklyn Botanical Gardens, an evening marathon of *Battlestar Galactica*, greeting a smiling friend at his door, her arms loaded with Stargazer lilies. Relive the first moment he played his thirty-pound baritone sax after chemo and radiation, reminding us that there's life after chemo.

In truth, for Fred, there was life during chemo. The essential Fred incarnates the meaning of what it means to be *present*. I witnessed countless moments where Fred conjured encouragement and humor for other patients and care providers with his alchemical ability to extract light from darkness, joy from horror, and defiance from defeat. Fred's staggering artistic legacy is rivaled only by his ability to expand time and space for everyone around him by the enormity of his *presence* to every moment of his life.

What is most striking about the diaries is their real-time quality and unabashed attention to the gruesome details of what it means to have colon cancer. Fred Ho is fighting a war, and as in any war, it is the details that bring us to understand the true nature of war. Contemporary mass media representations of war are sanitized and draped in the glories of heroism and flags presented to the wives and mothers of dead soldiers from their "grateful nation." We do not get to see the image of the soldier who must grip the rope of his intestines between his teeth to stop the bleeding, or the land mine–shattered bones jaggedly ripping through the tender flesh of a child's leg. We do not see the aftermath of post-traumatic stress disorder and its multigenerational metastasis.

It is not enough to invoke "the hell of war" or "the ravages of cancer"—we must feel the burn of bullets piercing skin; the blistering fevers; the stench of gangrene; the overflowing colostomy bag; the choking tumors, the ruptured throats; human organs floating in rivers, decaying in deserts, tossed into the formaldehyde jars of death's curio cabinet. Flags, medals, wigs, and prosthetics are not enough to convey the truth or mobilize human beings to dissent, resist, and demand the end of war, the cure for cancer, AIDS, and so many other mutant offspring of capitalism. It is not enough to hear the story of triumph and survival or sound the horn of victory. It is not enough to only see the faces of U.S. soldiers when we think of the dead; we must also see the dead among those we call the "enemy." The devil is not in the details, but in the absence of details that would activate the people to organize and demand greater efforts for the cures of disease, the end of war.

Finding cures to long-term diseases is not beneficial to the corporate pharmaceutical industry, just as peace would not benefit the military industrial complex. It is more profitable to extend an illness than to cure it, to extend a war than to end it. There is a killing field of silence spreading over the United States, a lethargy, a surrender to manufactured "realities" as we subjugate and opiate the true essence and reality of our own lives to the corporate media–manufactured, vicarious experience. We are afraid to look into the toilet of our existence, afraid to see that we have failed ourselves and future generations with silence, apathy, and the obsession with consumption. We have gone so far as to replace face-to-face communication with a language of convenience and speed—OMG!

Fred Ho's diaries slow us down, force us to engage multiple senses as he revivifies the violation of cancer in his body with straight talk. His raw courage and honesty snap us out of our collective malaise of social narcolepsy. Fred encourages us with humor, gratitude, and victories—both great and small. He teaches us that living fully is not always about being in a perfect state of health, but in a state of perfect presence to all our experiences, with or without cancer.

Three of the most significant weeks of my life were spent with Fred during his first surgery and subsequent recovery period. Sponge-bathing him in the hospital, avoiding the catheter, shaving his head, witnessing his vulnerability and the care and carelessness of health practitioners were not new experiences for me. Living these moments with someone like Fred, however, was inspiring. Fred remained his own vocal and ferocious advocate throughout the entire ordeal, even during times when a whisper was all he could muster. He granted friends, whom he refers to as his "cancer warriors," permission to speak on his behalf when the moment called for it. He dubbed me "The Enforcer" when it was time to challenge hospital staff. I still laugh when I think of the nurse who was offended by his choice to be nude in the stifling heat of an unventilated hospital room. Fred wanted to keep oxygen flowing through his extensive and wide surgical wound, preventing the growth of anaerobic bacteria, which could create a potentially life-threatening infection. Rage and humor filled us both at the thought that a nurse would be rattled by the sight of a nude human body. I politely invoked the Patient's Bill of Rights and requested that she not be allowed to attend to Fred again. Prudery can have lethal consequences, a fact that the history of tyranny confirms.

Fred's diaries are full of such details and moments of irony, pathos, and humor. These pages are loaded with lessons for self-advocacy and the importance of being an engaged patient with allies and witnesses. This book is about a journey of healing, which embraces the whole human being, and does not just focus on the cure. The cure is a crap shoot; healing is a process that integrates all aspects of the human being known as "the patient." Many glorious moments occur in a healing "process" that are ultimately the foundation of all recovery from any illness or dis-ease. At the very least, if the prognosis is finite, then let us allow the journey to be as life enriching as possible. Fred Ho is nobody's patient or a number on a chart. By the time he is done, he is nobody's honey or sweetie either. He is Mr. Ho, fighting for his life. Naked Fred. Take it or leave it.

When we returned to Fred's home, it was my task to clean and pack the oozing nine-inch open surgical wound that spanned from upper to lower abdomen. At first I was afraid, not of the wound, but of making an error that could lead to infection. This never happened. What did happen was that I had to face his suffering, my fear of doing harm by error, and the knowledge that this man, who is closer to me than a brother, might have a premature death. We talked about death, but mostly we enjoyed life. We shared stories, watched movies, listened to music, debated, argued, and laughed more than would seem possible; yes, stitches popped!

That horrible, beautiful wound was the landscape of our most significant meeting. More than performing or traveling together, more than any collaboration we had previously shared, that scary open wound offered us the gift of understanding the profoundest meaning of friendship, underscoring for us both; what most matters in life is not our accomplishments, titles, awards or possessions, but the essence of living an entire lifetime with every breath—unconditional love, the undefeated champion of every revolution.

Take your own journey with Fred through this diary and be reminded to *live now,* because *living now* is better for your immune system than putting it off. Live, breathe, laugh, and get practical advice from a warrior with a good story to tell and the will to tell it.

May this book leave you breathless so that you may learn to breathe again.

MAGDALENA GÓMEZ

"Song from the Womb of Yemaya"
For Fred Ho, November 27, 2007

you carry the whale and dolphin inside you
sometimes they carry you.
in your body is a vast and pristine ocean
purity itself, fresh and sacred
it is washing away all that is not born of love
in your body there is only room for love
in your body there is only room for what is born of love
in your body there is only room for laughter
in your body there is only room for joyous memory
in your body there are ancient ocean friends and warriors
every dolphin and every whale
with whom you have shared a moment
remembers you and fights beside you;
when you are tired they fight on your behalf.
in your body there is only room for what is born of love
in your body there is only room for what is born of love
you are a dolphin
you are a whale
you are a vast and pristine ocean;
the sea grass lift sherdancing arms
holding up the harsh days to come
filling herself with all your struggles
you will not carry them alone;

the mermaids all know you by name
they blush remembering
your naked, liberated body
they laugh with joy and sacred sensual memory,
whispering to you:
in your body there is only room for what is born of love
in your body there is only room for what is born of love
you are a vast and pristine ocean
washing itself clean, fresh, whole, alive

moving through each moment with infinite wisdom
knowing that in your body there is only room
for what is born of love
in your body there is only room for what
is born of love.

MAGDALENA GÓMEZ

INTRODUCTION

THE ART OF BREATHING AND OTHER EVERYDAY REVOLUTIONARY PRACTICES

Breathing was already on my mind when I first met Fred Ho. Its beauty and banality, its strength and vulnerability, its simplicity and complexity, its unthinking ease and effortlessness, its ethereal materiality. Fred had invited me to a concert in a Soho loft, where his friend, sax player Earl Howard, melded his instrument with the strange and lovely vocalizations of Thomas Buckner. During the performance, sax and human voice met and intermingled until you could not tell which was which, and it was all about breath and its sublime possibilities to create beauty and community, and how unmistakably inseparable breath is from spirit, mind, and body.

I had been thinking about breathing because I had just seen an extraordinary film, *O Sopro Criando* by Brazilian artist Ernesto Neto, at the Park Avenue Armory. In the video, through his breathing on white talclike powder that covers a metal table, Neto blows a whole new geography into being—a lunarlike white landscape that, as it unfolds, is accompanied by the in-and-out staccato sound of the artist's labored breathing that brings this delicate world into being. I had also just finished reading Fred's *Diary of a Radical Cancer Warrior*, with its profoundly moving insights about the life-giving art of oxygenation. And I had been listening to his CD, *Celestial Green Monster*, where

Fred's sax gives exuberant testimony to Fred as a cancer warrior who not only is still breathing but also continuing to turn something as basic as breathing into an art form that brings people together. As Fred puts this in Diary, "I listen to my breath and to the music of others, to the breath of many others." These words resonated with me as I sat at this Soho performance, and I could not take for granted the sound of Fred's breathing nor could I understand it apart from the crafted explosions of breath that make music and other mindful manifestations of art.

Oxygenation constitutes one of the five crucial components in Fred Ho's war on cancer. In *Diary*, Fred describes coming to know breathing as a spiritual practice as well as evidence of being alive. He becomes ever more mindful of taking deep breaths, allowing for breathers, clearing the air, playing his sax, surrounding himself with plants and their oxidizing powers, and undergoing ozone infusions. The other key weapons in his arsenal—hydration, nutrition, self-healing, and *love*—are equally and indisputably foundational to survival. And, as *Diary* makes clear, to survive cancer requires going to war not only against the cancer itself but also against the capitalist order, the matrix that breeds and spreads cancer and other malignant conditions at the macro and micro levels, invading our very cells.

One of the most profound lessons of *Diary* is that, quite literally, change must happen at the cellular level. To revolutionize society and to combat cancer (and the two as Fred Ho shows us are inextricable) require attention to and restructuring of the cells that comprise individual living bodies and that connect these bodies to one another and to the living, breathing world around us. To shift away from capitalism and the cancer that is its monstrous creation requires a reconfiguration of cells. Fred Ho calls for nothing less in *Diary*. Through its daily details, *Diary* provides a blueprint for achieving such change. The plan of action, because it is one that individuals can implement through everyday actions and choices, is truly revolutionary. Here is a model for revolution that depends not upon violence (although Fred is no pacifist) or dramatic once-off upendings of the system, but rather upon daily acts of love and everyday uncompromisingly anticapitalist practices that create change at the cellular level and spread from there, a counter to a cancerous society.

Fred's road to revolution did not begin with his cancer diagnosis, but traces back through his early years. His commitment to fighting capitalism and its multiple and interlocking forms of oppression can be seen in his decades of political organizing with Asian Americans and immigrant communities, Marxist-Leninists, and radical people of color; in the music he produces, composes, and performs solo and with other Asian and African American musicians; in his writings; in his opposition to domestic violence; in his engineering of his own media labels; in his relationships and the daily ways in which he lives his life.

Fred Ho was born in 1957 in Palo Alto, California, to parents who both had immigrated to the United States from China. His father taught political science at the University of Massachusetts Amherst until 1987; his mother was a housewife who divorced Fred's father in 1988, after a ten-year battle with domestic violence—an experience that contributed to Fred's work to end violence against women (see his *Home Is Where the Violence Is*). Fred attended Harvard University, where he overcame his experience of alienation through various political awakenings. He immersed himself in campus and community organizing, including contending Marxist-Leninist organizations. He joined the Nation of Islam in 1975. His move off campus late in his freshman year to the Chinese immigrant section of the South End of Boston put him in contact with an older group of Asian American radicals, including members of the revolutionary group I Wor Kuen (Fred documents IWK's contributions in his edited collection, *Legacy to Liberation*). Fred became active in Asian American organizing both on and off campus. Fred also developed during this period as a musician: a musician during high school, he began taking classes and performing with Archie Shepp and other luminaries of the Black Arts Movement; and while in college, he did a brief stint with the Harvard jazz big band. Fred Ho graduated from Harvard as a Marxist-Leninist and as a musician intent on creating a new Asian American art form, and these commitments have remained constants through his many personal transformations. Indeed in 2009, Harvard University awarded him the Harvard Arts Medal, given to an alumnus who has distinguished him- or herself in the arts. Fred joined the I Wor Kuen in 1977 and worked construction. He developed cultural programs in Boston Chinatown including an immigrant and American-born Chinese folksong ensemble. In 1981, he moved to New York City to become a professional musician. Soon after he began traveling regularly to the San Francisco Bay Area to collaborate with pianist Jon Jang and other Asian American artist-activists. After disagreements with the League of Revolutionary Struggle (LRS) leadership that resulted in his being kicked out of the organization in 1989, Fred moved from his Manhattan loft to Brooklyn and plunged more deeply into the study of Marxism and intensified his artistic and political direction. By 1990, he was supporting himself as an artist and living in an upscale duplex loft in Park Slope. However, as Fred describes it, the toll of the mortgage and work stresses, combined with an unhealthy diet and growing personal ego, anger, and competitiveness made this a very carcinogenic period of seeking "more"—more success, more sex, more recognition—even as he also was continuing to lead Marxist study groups, support political prisoners, and innovate martial arts music/theater productions and other radical projects.

In 2000, Fred decided to downsize his life. He sold 70 percent of his material belongings and his duplex and bought a much more modest place in Greenpoint, Brooklyn. These decisions bought him greater artistic freedom—including the ability to subsidize his label Big Red Media, under which he produces avant-garde Afro Asian multicultural CDs (including *Big Red!*; *Year of the Tiger*; *Celestial Green Monster*; *Red Arc: A Call For Revolucion Con Salsa Y Cool*; *Voice of the Dragon: Once Upon a Time in Chinese America*; *Night Vision: A New First to Third World Opera*; *Turn Pain into Power*; *The Underground Railroad to My Heart*; *We Refuse to Be Used and Abused!*; *Tomorrow Is Now!*), DVDs (*The Black Panther Suite*), the manga/double-book CD project, *Deadly She-Wolf Assassin at Armageddon!/Momma's Song*, and calendars (Sheroes/Women Warrior Calendar). He also distributes his books (including *Legacy to Liberation* and *Wicked Theory, Naked Practice*) through Big Red Media. At once simplifying and taking greater charge of his own life also gave him the freedom to travel more for pleasure and to make of his home a sanctuary. Despite all these positive life changes, along with the joy of reuniting with the love of his life in April 2006, Fred continued to feel internally toxified and still on the treadmill—as a result, he began experiencing serious intestinal problems. In August 2006, he learned he had colorectal cancer. And in the course of fighting the cancer, a new Fred Ho was born. The *Diary* chronicles the emergence and continuing evolution of this Fred Ho.

Fred Ho's new sense of self emerges from a set of tactics and strategies that he devises to continue his ongoing war on capitalism and his struggles with cancer and the Capitalist Industrial Medical Establishment (CIME), capitalism's malignant by-products. *Diary* documents the development of these tactics and strategies, which draw on martial arts and Chinese medicine and which are informed by his beliefs in Ludditism, matriarchy, and Marxism. In keeping with Fred Ho's Marxist commitments, which have remained constant as he has gone through various transformations, I offer nine theses that I have derived from *Diary*.

1. The warrior fighting cancer also must wage a war against capitalism.

Diary blows apart the common perception that the answer to curing cancer lies in research for better treatments or more affordable drugs. Although discovering treatments and making them universally accessible are indispensable, they do not reach the root of the problem: "The death of cancer," Fred states, "will only come about when the very conditions of toxicity that give growth to cancer cells have been eliminated. What we are faced with it is how systemic the conditions of toxicity are: engendered and enhanced by all the 'things' that are accepted as 'natural' to capitalist-industrial society." As long as there is capitalism and its far-reaching forms of toxicity, there will be cancer. As *Diary* makes clear, cancer cannot be understood apart from capitalism, a system that views everything and everyone only in terms of the profits they generate, and creates an emotionally and environmentally toxic world that makes people—and all living things—sick. In large part, this is because illness is big business in the United States, especially for pharmaceutical corporations and insurance companies. Under capitalism, even cancer becomes a moneymaking enterprise, and many of the same corporations that develop cancer drugs pollute the environment with cancer-creating toxins. Not only are we constantly exposed to the increasing number of carcinogens in our food, in the air we breathe, and in all that surrounds us, but also the pressures and imbalances of scrambling for more money and more material markers of success render people even more vulnerable to incurring cancer. Thus, Fred's insight in *Diary* that cancer like capitalism is experienced and must be fought at the cellular level. Fighting cancer, Fred explains, "is a war fought on the medical/cellular level, it is a war fought on the social-economic-political level against the U.S. HMO system of profiteering off health care, and it is a war fought on the spiritual-physical-mental-manual level of yin yang."

As Fred Ho comes increasingly to believe, allopathic or mainstream medicine itself has left humans behind, caught up as it is in the pursuit of profits and the institutional arrogance that accompany capitalism. His later entries chronicle his increasing awareness of ways medical professionals have bought into the Capitalist Industrial Medical Establishment. "The CIME doctors and staff," Fred finds, "are prisoners of their paradigm, protocols and the profit-driven system." Fred's "no-compromise" turn to self-healing is at once a rejection of a capitalist economy and the havoc it wreaks on individual and social bodies, and an embrace of an alternative economy founded upon collective well-being, beauty, creativity, and caring.

2. The struggle against cancer requires acknowledge of, not shame for, the havoc the disease wreaks on one's body.

In *Diary*, Fred refuses to sanitize the body or the experience of cancer. As he makes clear, cancer and its treatments involve blood and pus and shit, rashes, zits, hair loss, weight gain, weight loss, inability to sustain an erection, and other painful indignities. Parts of *Diary* are so graphic that they are difficult to read, but in telling the truths of his body in agonizing detail, Fred does battle with social niceties, which would have us deny or mask the force of our bodies and which lead many of us to experience shame or a loss of self-esteem when our bodies escape our control or defy social norms. When Fred describes day after day of diarrhea and how he is held hostage to his bowels in a way that strips him of his ability to eat or sleep or control where he shits, his account of these torturous realities is a generous one; it destigmatizes loss of bodily control as it lets others with cancer know what they might expect. Fred does not candy-coat the severe depression that can attend such physical agony and inability to master one's most basic bodily functions. Mind, spirit, and body—*Diary* demonstrates time and again—are connected. And although there are ways we are inevitably alone in experiencing illness, for those undergoing experiences similar to Fred's, he provides knowledge that they aren't the only ones, and he gives license to discuss—and so lacerates—the blistering wounds that silence can create. For those who might not be undergoing such experiences but have loved ones who are, his narrative enables them to better understand and help those for whom they care.

3. When you mindfully care for your body, you also feed your soul and create possibilities for social transformation.

Fred's main tenets in *Diary* relate to ways to help your body fight cancer that are as basic as they are profound in their implications for spiritual-well being and societal health.

For Fred, oxygenation is imperative in fighting cancer. And as he describes it in *Diary*, breathing is elemental to life and art, but is no simple matter. Breathing is not only evidence of being alive:"To breathe deeply daily and to *listen* to one's breath is to feel and 'hear' one's soul." Although breathing is automatic, mindful breathing is meditation, is art inducing, is pain relieving, is life giving, is communion with others, is critical perspective on and escape from the moneymaking treadmill. In *Diary*, when Fred says he is "fighting with every breath in my body to bring an end to the capitalist system," he means this quite literally.

Water, too, is an elemental and life-giving force. Water is increasingly privatized and polluted in today's economy. Water also is basic to survival, whether it be the water that you drink or the water in which you bathe or swim to cleanse your body and spirit. Fred insists throughout *Diary* on the need to stay hydrated with filtered water. *Diary* also conjures up the ocean and the peacefulness and joy that immersion in it brings. Appreciation for pure water's power to rejuvenate the body and spirit means caring for the land and sea over and above the profits that can be extracted from them.

Eating well is also essential to countering both capitalism and cancer. *Diary* gives its readers detailed information about how to eat well (where to shop, what kind of foods to eat and how to prepare them, when to eat) and what foods best fight cancer. Fred explains his conviction that a bad diet—that lots of barbequed meats and other chemically laden, high-fat, hydrogenated, and carcinogenic foods—contributed significantly to his contracting cancer, and *Diary* documents his increasing awareness that a diet of fish and fresh fruits and vegetables, organic and locally grown and prepared with minimal or no cooking, not only help the body to fight cancer but are also a means for us all to remain as healthy as possible in a world where the relentless quest for profits pollutes our food and water. Eating well, in other words, provides a challenge to the capitalist structures that breed cancer.

To the less-than-attentive reader, the extensive and detailed entries about Fred's diet might seem extraneous—ones that can be skimmed or skipped. However, they make up a crucial ingredient of *Diary*. Implementing the kind of eating regime that Fred lays out not only serves as a means for resisting cancer but also a more general plan for overall health and well-being that simultaneously chips away at corporate structures: because locally grown and organic foods tend to be produced by small business owners or by more environmentally minded companies, eating well tends also to be a daily way to be less complicit in the corporate practices that spread toxicity.

As *Diary* progresses, Fred's eating practices become evermore resistant to and undermining of a capitalist economy. In the fall of 2010, when his cancer recurs for the fourth time, Fred decides to fight it with a raw food diet rather than following his doctors' plan to remove his rectum, despite their acknowledgment that this drastic surgery might not prove curative. The no-compromise manifesto that Fred devises in response to his cancer's recurrence includes the adoption of a raw food diet. The last entries to *Diary* describe Fred's diet and its dramatic benefits to him physically, emotionally, and spiritually.

As is absolutely characteristic of Fred, this attention to diet is as profoundly political as it is personal. Going raw is part of his conviction that Malcolm X was right when he proclaimed, "Revolution is extremism." A raw food diet puts into practice his advocacy for self-sufficient food production that can replace agribusiness industrial food production. It is a means to stop planetary degradation and cancerous toxicity. Accompanying Fred's movement to adopt a raw food diet is his work at a collectively run farm where he is involved in growing his own food. Farming and living off the fruits of one's labor build health at the individual and societal level in a number of ways. Growing and harvesting food involves physical exercise and engenders connectedness to the earth. In addition, eating local produce is more healthful—fruits and vegetables are not shot through with chemicals used to grow and preserve them in transit as they are shipped far from their point of origin. Moreover, farming, as practiced by Fred, is a collective, community-building enterprise, and one that provides an alternative to a for-profit economy.

In *Diary*, eating well builds a deeply nourishing political community not just in the process of producing food, but also in the making and eating of it. Food's health-giving properties increase when it is prepared by and shared with friends and family—when it is made with love and consumed with loved ones. Fred's comprehensive accounts of who cooks for him, and of the details of each dish, evidence the powers of food to bring emotional and spiritual as well as physical well-being, and provide a life-sustaining model for community. The Raw Fight Club he organizes not only provides him with companionship but also is part of his and his comrades' "efforts toward constructing new social relations free from the cash-nexus, emancipatory from capitalism." The Raw Fight Club is but the latest manifestation of Fred's understanding that "if spirituality is to matter, then it must be materialist."

4. You cannot fight cancer on your own: independence is an undesirable fiction.

One of the revolutionary things about *Diary* is that it refuses the masculinist myth of self-sufficiency and bourgeois individualism and offers a model that opposes its pathologies. Too often, not only in the dominant culture but also in more progressive subcultures, being a man means asserting one's autonomy, however illusory, since independence is invariably underwritten by various forms of erased or invisible labor. Theorists in disability and feminist studies have done a good job establishing the harmful consequences of the myth that humans are, or should be, independent, autonomous beings. One ill effect of this myth is that society is structured not for universal accommodation but with the assumption that we are all able-bodied and independent. Curb cuts provide a simple illustration of this: rather than rounded curbs that are accessible to those in wheelchairs or pushing children in strollers, the norm until recently has been curbs cut at right angles. Activists and scholars in feminist and disability studies also have pointed out that although living with a disability puts our forms of dependency into sharp relief, we are *all* vulnerable and depend on one another, although for the able-bodied, and for men in particular, this reality is often obscured, and to ill effect for all.

Fred debunks this ideology through his willingness to ask for the help that he needs, and for his unfailing recognition of—and deep appreciation for—the loving assistance he receives. *Diary* contains a record of the individuals who have contributed in a variety of ways to Fred's survival and well-being. Drivers, cooks, companions, caretakers, housekeepers—those who send or bring gifts or offer medical or legal advice are all acknowledged and thanked. In this way, Fred challenges the prevailing social order, one in which caretakers, in particular, who are disproportionately women, often engage in work—whether paid or unpaid—that goes unmentioned and is disrespected and undervalued. Rather than hide or obscure his dependence, or feel emasculated by it, Fred lays bare his dependency on others. He renders visible the kinds of labor on which to varying degrees we all, whether ill or not, depend.

In *Diary*, dependence is not at odds with self-advocacy (a necessity when navigating the complexities of the medical system) or with the self-healing that Fred comes to embrace when his cancer recurs for the fourth time. Self-healing for Fred does not mean going it alone, but rather refusing to give his life over to a medical institution that has disrespected and dehumanized him. Self-healing entails charting his own journey, but seeing that as he undertakes it, he does so accompanied by those he loves and trusts—Dr. Bill Akpinar, his Raw Fight Club, his family, and his friends. Fred Ho makes clear that such dependency is a strength rather than a weakness, because it enables survival and the pleasures that come with being part of a network of loving relationships. To "put a stare on cancer and dance it to death" requires the company of other dancer/warriors.

5. Cancer is best fought through a circle of love.

We live in a culture where when we ask, "Are you in a relationship?" we are asking if one is part of a romantic couple. If the answer is no, we say a person is single or alone, regardless of the webs of relationships in which one may be deeply enmeshed. Fred's *Diary* not only refuses the idea that one is single or alone if not part of a couple, but it testifies to the emotional richness and pleasures that attend finding nourishment through what Fred calls his circle of love. Fred's circle of love includes a range of relationships. His circle is made up of friends, many of whom are musicians or artists and/or political comrades; his lover; family members; and health professionals. Each has a role to play in his life, and the affectionate bonds that this circle of love creates enables Fred to find and embrace health, nourishment, companionship, beauty, friendship, art, and music. *Diary* was initially written to Fred's circle: it itself is a labor of love even as it testifies to the life-sustaining contributions of Fred's circle of love.

6. A circle of love offers an alternative to capitalist kinship structures.

Diary's model of community has far-reaching implications for thinking about anticapitalist alternatives to the nuclear family and the forms of class, sexual, and gender oppression it engenders. As we have learned from Marx, the nuclear family is an invention that underwrites a capitalist economy. One of its most basic if outdated and often deadly units, the nuclear family assumes a father who provides income that sustains the family and a mother who makes possible the father's labor by taking care of the home, the children, and her husband. The ways in which this model disempowers women have been well established. Under this arrangement, women are financially vulnerable and emotionally dependent upon men who undervalue their labor and view women as both prized possessions and as taken-for-granted sources of labor. For households in which women work (which now include middle- and upper middle-class families in addition to working-class and poor families), women often continue to assume all or a disproportionate share of the domestic duties. The rise in middle- and upper middle-class women who work has had particularly adverse effects on poor and working-class women, especially single mothers who are often unable to take care of their own homes and children, sometimes because they are being paid to take care of middle-class homes and children. The reigning assumption under the present set of arrangements, that one is either cared *for* or a care*taker*, creates a toxic imbalance. It leaves many women, who are most often the caretakers (whether paid or unpaid), materially dependent and emotionally depleted.

The inequities of this arrangement are heightened when disability is introduced into a household. If it is the caretaker who is disabled, who takes care of her? And if it is the breadwinner or children, the caretaker's labor often increases exponentially. As for the person being taken care of, his or her own dependency can have complex consequences that can include a disavowal of or need to assert control over the caretaker. This is perhaps especially true for men who are assumed to be more independent than women, and who, to negate their need for their caretakers, can assert tyrannical forms of control over them to bolster their own threatened sense of masculinity.

Fred's circle of love provides a salutary alternative to these cruel imbalances. The beauty of Fred's model is that it is fuelled by love rather than capital. And the communal structure of Fred's circle of love escapes the claustrophobia, the inequitable burdens, and the exploitation that structure the heteronormative social organization created under capitalism. In Fred's circle of love, we find a structure wherein caretaking is spread out and becomes a source of pleasure and reciprocity. No one person is sucked dry emotionally or materially, and each can give what she or he is able to and desires. Fred's circle of love therefore escapes the forms of material exploitation and emotional abuse that are inherent to the dominant system in place in our society today. Thus the structure Fred establishes through recounting the daily acts of care from members of his circle of love is not simply a quotidian account of how he organizes his life: it also embodies a Marxist feminist vision that has something to offer every person, whether or not they are experiencing an illness or disability.

7. To survive and thrive means to let go of attachments to ego.
Fred's openness to others and to the care and love they offer him and his disavowal of competition and ambition to succeed in the terms of the dominant culture are all connected to Fred's letting go of ego. As Fred discovers through the course of *Diary*, to view the self as supreme is to be caught up in an economy in which a successful individual is selfish, overrun by ego, and insatiable in the quest for more money and possessions and other markers of status. To be caught up in such a system, Fred explains, can all too readily result in cancer. To let go of ego is to rid the body of toxicity and to create a healthier world. If each of us were to let go of ego, capitalism would come to a grinding halt and in its place would be an economy governed by love and concern for others. Such a vision is of course a utopian one, and what such a world would look like is difficult to imagine, but Fred suggests that to strive for such a world is far from a luxury, nor is it a vision to give up on. To create this kind of change, one must exercise humility and openness to change, maintain an optimism of the will, and a willingness to move step by step. What *Diary* chronicles is just such a series of movements.

8. Revolution—overturning capitalism and cancer—is a set of daily practices and not a singular event.
Being ill heightens and lays bare the cancerous structures in which we are all implicated. *Diary* therefore not only provides assistance and inspiration to those struggling with cancer, but it also offers a revolutionary blueprint for all readers. The daily nature of the diary is the perfect vehicle for forwarding a model of change that is incremental and achievable by altering one's most ordinary practices. If effecting such change is possible, it is also difficult and requires discipline, vision,

and imagination. "To paraphrase Sun Tzu," Fred writes in *Diary*, "conquering is easy, transforming is hard." In *Diary*, one does not go to war against cancer and capitalism through large and violent actions, but through daily practices of hydration, oxygenation, nutrition, self-healing, and love that are at once extreme and extremely doable. Certainly, if exercised at the individual level, these practices will result in greater health and happiness. But if these practices spread and become collective ones, they become antibodies that can attack the cancerous creature that goes by the name of capitalism. As Fred Ho exhorts, "Yes, change begins with the individual, indeed at the cellular level, and if it is to be real and genuine, insistently at the cellular and must extend far beyond the individual into the social and engage the entire universe."

9. The point, in other words, is for us to change the world, cell by cell. These steps will help to take us there!

As I hope these theses suggest, *Diary* is no purely personal quotidian account of cancer. Part theory, part manifesto, part instruction manual, part tribute to Fred Ho's circle of love, *Diary* offers a radical vision for change. In its deeply political nature and in its revolutionary impetus, *Diary* resembles another autobiographical narrative, just as Fred himself resembles its author, another intellectual and visionary revolutionary. I am thinking, of course, of *The Autobiography of Malcolm X* and of Malcolm X himself.

Like Malcolm X, what characterizes Fred is a radical openness, an insistence of "by any means necessary" and an understanding that the means will change, and as they do, the self will be transformed, again and again. Even as Fred Ho offers *Diary* as an account of rebirth, what strikes me about Fred Ho is how, like Malcolm X, he maintains a combination of fierce, absolutely constant, and uncompromising commitment to overturning oppression at the same time as he remains open to radical change and self-transformation. These men also share their fearlessness in speaking the truth as they see it, and both are constitutionally incapable of selling out. Fred Ho, like Malcolm X, has not only an unwavering opposition to injustice but also the radical openness and thirst for knowledge that gives him the courage to re-create himself in his revolutionary journey.

What you hold in your hands is an account of this ongoing journey, and its lessons. Take a deep breath and read on. May *Diary of a Radical Cancer Warrior: Fighting Cancer and Capitalism at the Cellular Level* be as radically transformative for you as the fight against cancer has been for Fred Ho.

CYNTHIA G. FRANKLIN

Prologue

I AM NOT A CANCER SURVIVOR BUT A CANCER FIGHTER!

I dislike and oppose the term "cancer survivor." "Survivors" implies those who somehow, favored or fated by miracle (or luck), escaped the massive fatalities of a great evil or enemy (such as Holocaust survivors). Fascism is the most aggressive and militarized manifestation of capitalism (bourgeois dictatorship), the complete abrogation of any democratic political pretense for outright state-military governance.

My friend, woodsman Jay Crotchett, pointed out that cancer and capitalism are the same processes of accelerated, aggressive malignant growth. Taking Jay's analysis, fascism is capitalism at its most malignant and aggressive stage. Cancer is the culmination of carcinogenic activity in which normal processes of one's immune system have become overwhelmed and veritably "consumed" or conquered by malignancy.

Instead of "cancer survivor" I prefer "cancer fighter" or "cancer warrior." Because the precise or predominant causes of cancer remain uncertain to the allopathic paradigm and, in my belief, will remain unexplainable to that paradigm because the "causes" are inextricable from the very genesis and development of modern capitalist existence, why one person "survives" or another doesn't cannot equally be ascribed. For now, given our understanding of both the disease and its interaction with "the system" of modern industrial capitalist existence, since who *survives* and who doesn't cannot be predicted or sufficiently explained, then the only recourse for the cancer patient is to fight. For the person still cancer free, fighting cancer also becomes imperative rather than "hoping" to avoid it, taking preventive and prepared measures to undermine it (since cancer and capitalism in my thesis grow together, it cannot be preempted, only eliminated simultaneously).

In the recognition of the alarming growth of cancer rates, especially in affluent societies, it is perhaps an almost commonsensical acknowledgment that "it's not a matter of if one will get cancer, but when." (At one point, the most primitive human societies, such as the nomadic Kalahari bush people, evinced no modern diseases such as cancer, heart disease, or diabetes. That, however, as globalization has touched every inch of this biosphere, is no longer true. I am told that the only places where cancer rates have dropped to near zero are societies encountering mass starvation, such as Darfur or among the Jews imprisoned during World War II in fascist concentration camps.)

Even if five or ten years from now I appear to be cancer free—for however long I will live on this planet—I am both obligated and committed to continue to be a cancer warrior. But as the pages of my cancer war diary will attest, there are no lone warriors, no single struggle waged by a heroic individual, but a circle of people who have chosen to join the "Warriors for Fred" society. Without these friends and family members—these generous, brave, loyal, and dedicated warriors—I most likely would not have survived. They have been the sustenance for the struggle, providing logistical, moral, spiritual, financial, and medical support for me. They are the front and rear guard forces in the general war against this deadly evil. They are the warriors against the greatest killer of all time. (In America alone over fifty thousand people a year are killed by colorectal cancer.)

HOW THE WAR BEGAN

I was officially diagnosed with stage 3b colorectal cancer on August 4, 2006, after a colonoscopy was performed on me. I was about to turn forty-nine years old. The American Cancer Society and mainstream U.S. medicine strongly recommends men to have regular colonoscopies after turning fifty. I went because I was having constant diarrhea, and stool test results were all negative for any viral causes (I was assuming I had caught some "bug" from my constant travels to the third world, including Egypt, the Dominican Republic, Columbia, Cambodia, and Thailand within the past year). The size of the tumor was very large, about the size of a golf ball, blocking my colon tract and forcing my waste matter to be compressed into liquid in order to evacuate.

Because of the size, which my sister, who was at that time a physician and researcher at the Food and Drug Administration, believed that the tumor had been growing inside of me for about ten years, I had to undergo immediate surgery to remove the tumor, which was performed on August 25, 2006. I was "staged" at 3b (stage 1 is small tumor, stage 4 is almost certain death as only 8 percent of people at stage 4 survive). Given the size of the tumor, the biopsy also showed that one out of twenty-two lymph nodes removed were positive for cancer, and that the disease had broken through my perineum.

THE WARRIOR SISTERS GET ORGANIZED

While recovering from surgery, I knew I had to undergo chemotherapy treatment within six weeks. Given the urgency and limited time, a core of close friends organized themselves to provide whatever support I needed, including transportation, companionship and assistance for doctors' visits and chemo treatments, food shoppers and deliverers, visitors to look in on me and help with household and daily living chores. One friend, Bob Lederer, came up with the idea of a LISTSERV called "Warriors for Fred," to keep my many friends across the world informed of the war I am fighting against cancer. People who wanted to know how I am doing, how they can help, would request to join the Warriors list and be informed of the war, what I needed, and how they could be marshaled into specific support activity. My core team included Ann T. Greene (whom I refer to as my "general" for her leadership and administrative role), Magdalena Gómez (whom I refer to as my "sergeant major" who performs much of the day-to-day groundwork), Paget Walker, and Jennifer Feil. Many other friends, too numerous to list here, all stepped forward to take on many responsibilities.

One of the women warriors who soon joined our army, Peggy Choy, admonished me for using patriarchal military ranking and admonished me to use terms such as "warrior queens." I agree with Peggy's proposed matriarchal military conception, with the one caveat that Ann T. Greene still be recognized as the "general" (in the vein of the character Ashanti Nana (Queen Mother) Ya Asantewa in the opera Ann and I co-created, *Warrior Sisters: The New Adventures of African and Asian Women Warriors* about a decade ago).

I decided to write regular blog entries to the LISTSERV, which have resulted in this journal titled *Diary of a Radical Cancer Warrior: Fighting Cancer and Capitalism at the Cellular Level.* The diary method has been used by all of the great martial artists to unite strategy, tactics, and to develop a deeper philosophical and theoretical exploration of methods and experiences in protracted fighting. It is hoped that all who read the *Diary* entries will understand that cancer and capitalism are inextricable and that no possible *cure* can be found so long as the toxicity of capitalist existence continues. And more profoundly, that it can be fought and eventually defeated if correct analysis and methods of combat are applied.

THE WAR RETURNS

My initial chemo treatments ended March 10, 2007. On September 25, 2007, my annual colonoscopy revealed that the tumor had returned. An MRI subsequently revealed another possible tumor in my pelvic region. The war did not end, but continued. I underwent a combination of different chemotherapy treatments with radiation, which finished the end of January 2008. I would have another surgery, have an ileostomy bag attached to me, undergo even more chemotherapy, surgical removal of the bag and a gaping "crater" in my upper right abdomen, proceed to fly to Madison, Wisconsin, to begin a artist teaching residency within two weeks after leaving the hospital with an undetermined life-threatening fever that reached 104 degrees, and, in December 2008, to have a colonoscopy that once again found cancer cells.

GOD HAS SOMETHING MORE TO TEACH ME

This is what my friend Mike Surdej told me—it was the only explanation he could come up with as many cancer patients have tormented themselves with the question, Why me? In war, collateral damage is massive, and to ask the question, Why me? Is a misplacement of energy and focus. Rather, to acknowledge the state of siege or war and proceed to fight to end it must be the predominant effort. I often tell young people that the best way for me to learn has been to get my ass kicked and that my role as a teacher is to kick their asses. Well, getting cancer has been a massive ass kicking for me that has taught me much. In the diary, I outline both the physical losses (perhaps likely to be permanent) but more importantly, the philosophical gains. Many of these gains could not have come any other way but through this harsh, brutal, dangerous war. My conceptions about Ludditism, getting off "the treadmill," of love, about a new vision of the revolutionary struggle, the journey to eliminate ego, my mission on this planet, my preparedness to die, to live fighting with every breath in my body to bring an end to the capitalist system. All these radical and new conceptions are all detailed within the diary: how they were sparked, developed, and transformed me.

As a real-time instructional war diary and manual, my struggle has no neat or final ending, and until my death, whether it be soon or extended to be later (as of publication, I am still alive and fighting!), may never have a definitive conclusion. When I submitted the initial manuscript for this war diary to Skyhorse Publishing, I had believed that I was in remission, and wrote an afterword, contained herein, that expressed this then-apparent conclusion.

However, cancer would return a fourth time, diagnosed early fall 2010, and would pose new challenges and a major change in direction for the New Fred Ho with the complete rejection of four years of the allopathic paradigm, to be replaced by a naturopathic paradigm for which, to date, I am currently pursuing with full commitment.

That is why this *Diary* is in two parts. It may disturb and shock some readers hoping to find a clear and effective solution relying upon the allopathic model. I have found none, after committing to it with intensity (being what my friend, Dr. Joseph Harris, described me as being "the perfect cancer patient" for the mainstream medical establishment). True to my radical beliefs and convictions, I am on my current journey to find a naturopathic solution, one that upholds my personal dignity and quality of life above all else, including life itself, to be in command of my decisions and thereby never accept compromises with the capitalist medical industry.

For readers trying to understand either their personal war against cancer, or of their friends or loved ones, this is not a simple or easy story. It is a story of unremitting struggle against terrible forces: capitalism, which is the cancer for Planet Earth; and cancer, which is the exponentially increasing environmental and social toxicity of capitalism assaulting the individual person.

Make no mistake: this is a war to the end, an end to which success or failure depends on how much we make ourselves to be the principled warriors in seeking solutions and not compromises to our personal health, wellness, transformation, and to curing the planet once and for all of the greatest threat to life itself.

Part One:
The Cancer War Begins

PLEASE JOIN THE "WARRIORS FOR FRED" LISTSERV BY EMAILING MAGDALENA GÓMEZ. YOU WILL RECEIVE WEEKLY UPDATES, HAVE ACCESS TO PHOTOS, AND DISCUSS WITH OTHER LISTSERV MEMBERS.

September 7, 2006

I was diagnosed with colon cancer on August 4, 2006, and had surgery to remove a very large malignant tumor on August 25, 2006. I was discharged to my apartment on August 31, 2006 where I am fighting to recover and prepare for the next stages of this battle. The pathology report has me at stage 3b—not good. There are 4 stages with 1 being most hopeful and 4 being terminal.

I decided only to inform a very small group of people who were willing and available to respect my privacy and do what had to be done to get me through the surgery and initial ambulatory period. Please forgive me if I did not inform you, but I am now home and reaching out to all of you.

September 20, 2006 (by Arthur Song)

Most of Fred's scar is healing well. He did have a bad allergic rash to the adhesive tape used to patch the sterile gauze to his abdomen, but alcohol cleaning and tea tree oil helped blast away the bacteria. His original two open holes—the largest being about 1.25 inches long, .75 inches wide, and .5 inches deep—became four holes sometime in week 2 possibly from Fred's overactivity and great amount of laughter that his friends instilled in him. These four holes now are very reduced in size, barely .125 inches deep, oozing a lot less blood and pus. Probably in two weeks they will be completely healed.

Every day Fred gets more strength and is more active. He hopes this week he can sit up for at least an hour by his table to begin copying parts out from the big band score he completed before going into surgery on August 25, 2006.

Fred is very grateful and appreciative of the wonderful times and foods all of you have contributed. Peter Adelman's fantastic chicken soup when Fred just got out of the hospital provided much-needed protein with savory flavor. Magdalena's constant vigilance, care, love, and cooking. The beautiful flowers brought weekly by Marina Celander and her contacting former cast members of Fred's productions. The great meal of salmon and potatoes by Gladys Serrano. Melanie's help and cooking. Taylor Ho Bynum's delicious Chinese kung pao chicken (without nuts!). Nikos Brisco's riotous DVDs. The vacuuming by David Bindman. The driving done by Jennifer, Paget, Ruth, Mark O'Ferrall, and Taylor to Fred's many doctors' appointments. General Ann T. Greene's administrative leadership. And the many people who have dropped by, brought food, done chores, and errands.

His nutrition must be high protein/low fat, low sodium, high antioxidants, and fiber (blueberries, salads, etc.). Note: All fresh produce should *not* be purchased from bodegas and places were produce sits piled in bins. Farmers' markets or refrigerated clean produce environments are important. Fish, Asian cooked tofu (not soy-processed products), chicken, some beef, and pork are good.

Nothing deep fried or greasy should be eaten. Fred loves sweet-and-sour pork, fried chicken, french fries, etc. *Do not* let him talk you into getting these things for him.

Of course, your good cheer, love, and friendship are very important so he doesn't feel isolated and can share his feelings about what he's going through.

We want to end this cancer once and for all now. We cannot afford a recurrence. If such a recurrence should happen, Fred will be in stage 4 (terminal, no recovery possible).

Your prayers, chants, thoughts are all welcome. You can drive, cook, drop by, and talk to Fred. You can join the Warriors for Fred LISTSERV to get regular updates and find out how you can help. Please respect Fred's wishes to be called only between 7:00 PM to 9:00 PM. He talks to everyone and always returns calls within twenty-four hours.

Once his open wound heals and his stomach is stronger, he will begin to swim and gently work out. He also hopes to be practicing the baritone saxophone again and to resume writing and composing and creating new shows.

Here is some background to this warrior's discipline and determination:

August 4, 2006, when malignant tumor was found, Fred weighed 218 pounds; blood pressure was 145/90.

August 25, 2006 when surgery was performed Fred, through swimming and hand-to-hand combat training, lowered his weight to 210 pounds; blood pressure was lowered to 120/80.

August 26, 2006, with the moral support of Nurse Anschel Hyacinthe, Fred pulls himself out his hospital bed and does three laps around the sixth floor. Every day from this point, he does these walks. He refuses to take any painkillers.

August 31, 2006 Fred returns home. His blood pressure is 120/80; his weight is 203 pounds.

September 20, 2006, at this report Fred weighs 200 pounds (lost 18 pounds since August 4); blood pressure is 110/70 (better than textbook numbers).

We want him to optimize his condition, his mental and physical strength for the next stage in this war.

September 26, 2006 (by Arthur Song)

A FUNNY STORY

A friend of Fred's named Jayne Cortez called him, and he explained that one possible side effect of his treatment is peripheral neuropathy, which varies from simple coldness, numbness, and tingling in the fingers and toes, to complete loss of dexterity. Fred's sister Florence had warned him that he might have to face a serious trade-off between living for another thirty-five years and losing his dexterity and becoming a mediocre musician. Jayne laughed and laughed and laughed. She said, "Fred, you will never be a mediocre musician. Even if you couldn't move at all, you would figure out a new way to play the saxophone that no one else would or could come up with!"

Also, great news: Fred finally found a clinical trial (C08) that is covered by his HMO (Health Plus of NYS Medicaid). It is at the Oncology Institute of the Long Island Jewish Medical Center.

There are many wonderful things about this facility and its staff. The chemo treatment room is like a spa, beautiful wood floors, comfortable chairs/beds, a TV and DVD player, free food and beverages, etc. Because this is a research clinical trial, there is a team of specialists supervising and monitoring Fred, along with stringent protocols to guard against side effects and mishaps.

Fred will be entered into a randomized lottery via computer to determine whether he will be in

Group 1: FOLFOX standard formulary regimen; or
Group 2: above PLUS Avastin experimental treatment.

Fred wants to get group 2, a 50/50, coin-toss chance. We will know by October 6, the closing date of the trial, what group he will have been selected for.

All of you who believe in chanting, prayers, etc. should put your maximum mojo into getting Fred into group 2.

Fred found this clinical trial on his own by spending countless hours searching via phone, Internet, and word of mouth. He has had to *hound* the system to get his records, etc. He is not lacking in diligence and determination, and he is appreciative and grateful to all the help, love, and emergency responses all his friends and warriors have given.

But this is a war. Winning battles doesn't mean the war will be won. But we will win if none of us accepts defeat, gets lax, or distracted. The war is expected to last ten years (the required length of his monitoring according to the clinical trial protocols). We expect to see many more new shows, performances, books, and good times between 2007 and 2017 from Fred Ho!

October 3, 2006 (by Arthur Song)

Fred Ho did *not* get randomized into Group 2 (the FOLFOX PLUS Avastin treatment in the clinical trial) as we were all praying, chanting, and hoping for. This means he got Group 1, the standard FOLFOX regimen.

However, he did travel today to Philadelphia to meet with a leading oncologist, Dr. Edith Mitchell, and learned several important things:

1. The clinical trials are required to begin chemo within seven days of registration. Fred was registered on September 27, 2006. This is why he is scheduled to begin, no matter what group, this Thursday, October 5, 2006.
2. The standard of quality care is that he should have chemo within forty-two days after surgery. He had surgery on August 25, 2006. Forty-two days later is October 6, 2006. The longer he delays, the more risk of cancer cells multiplying and thus spreading.
3. Once he begins any chemo treatment, he cannot enter any other clinical trials.
4. The greatest consideration Fred or any cancer patient should have is *not* the drug but the quality of *total* medical care, most especially important is the doctor's judgment and decision-making realm of experience and abilities. The doctor should be a specialist of colorectal cancer. Dr. Mitchell didn't think it wise to wage a five- to six-month battle with Medicaid and postpone any chemo until then. She also felt that she or any reputable and ethical physician couldn't argue for Avastin (or any drug, not FDA approved) unless some question/evidence of metastasis can be proven (meaning spread of cancer). It is for the following reasons:
   a. Avastin's side effects and proven-ness for below stage 4 cancer are still being studied, and no doctor would risk liability or the possible dangers or bear the cost if Fred's HMO won't cover the treatment of such side effects.
   b. A doctor who would accept cash payments (ranging from $50,000 to $250,000 plus other costs of side-effect treatment, etc.) is perhaps ethically suspect. The main consideration should

not be the money but the quality of care and decision-making capacities of the doctor.

c. Almost no doctor would administer Avastin, even if Fred could pay for it, without it being considered a tested and approved method whose advantages and efficacy clearly and demonstrably outweigh the side effects and risks, unless there is confidence that the drug can effectively counter widespread metastatic condition (which is the case for stage 4, but still being studied for the lower stages). This hasn't been proven; a drug like Avastin is still in the early-to-midway testing period.

Fred has decided to continue with the FOLFOX treatment at Long Island Jewish Medical Center for the following reasons:

1. The professional and high quality of the staff, doctors, and facility.
2. The incentive of being in a clinical trial in which everyone treating him *wants* his success.
3. The fact that the institution is a research and teaching facility offers a wider realm of experience, knowledge, and decision-making capacity.
4. The chemo treatment room is spacious and offers private patient treatment areas (not 20-plus people staring deathly into each other's faces with machines attached to them), along with a TV and DVD player, kitchen and beverages, and food.
5. The support staff wanting to get Fred Access-A-Ride and helping every way they can to ensure his highest quality of care and experience.

Should the possibility arise of obtaining Avastin or Erbitux (a.k.a. cetuximab, of the Martha Stewart Imclone scandal fame), Fred can consult and consider this addition, though he may have to leave the test.

So we will go into FOLFOX at Long Island Jewish Hospital.

Drivers are urgently needed for the first month of his visits for round-trip transportation and possible chemo partners to be with him. He needs to be taken home promptly and hooked up to a portable chemo pump by a visiting nurse who will be waiting for him at his building.

THINGS PEOPLE CAN DO IN NYC AND OUTSIDE NYC

1. Send noni juice, flaxseed oil, pomegranate juice. For example, a battalion of warriors in Hawaii are sending Fred organic noni juice.
2. Bring over planets and potted flowers (both medium and small size) for Fred's apartment to add beauty and extra *oxygen*!
3. Take Fred to the Bronx or Brooklyn Botanic Garden for several hours of oxygenation in the greenhouse. Oxygen is anticancer—cancer is antioxygen.
4. Help with driving and rides and perhaps visit with him while he is having chemo at the hospital or at his home.
5. Bring over oatmeal, juices, and other powerful antioxidants.
6. For those with institutional clout, Fred will need performing and speaking/teaching gigs in 2007 to make up for lost time and income—his band, the Afro Asian Music Ensemble, or Fred Ho as individual performer or speaker is available for bookings.
7. Be an emergency driver/contact person should at any time dangerous side effects occur and he needs to be taken immediately and directly to Long Island Jewish Medical Center. Please email for driving directions.

THINGS TO AVOID

1. People with children—as even the smallest cold may seriously harm Fred since his immune system will be wiped out.
2. Have Fred avoid public gatherings and public transportation where germs and the possibility of infection are magnified.
3. Fast foods, processed foods, high-temperature and oil-cooked foods, white sugars, white bread, dairy (except low-fat yogurt in smoothies or with flaxseed oil).

OCTOBER 5, 2006 (BY RUTH MARGRAFF WHO ACCOMPANIED FRED TO HIS FIRST DAY OF FOLFOX CHEMO TREATMENT AT LONG ISLAND JEWISH MEDICAL CENTER)

It was quite a scare yesterday afternoon at the chemo treatment. Toward 3:30 PM with the final injection (I believe this was the Decadron, but the nurses were not sure whether the reaction was a delayed reaction to the chemo or to this particular injection). Fred got very nauseous all of a sudden and his chest turned red (the red patch was almost like hives—he suddenly said he felt very hot and nauseous), and he was dozing off to unconsciousness.

The "push" or injection of the third treatment was immediately stopped. They gave Fred oxygen, Benadryl and something for antinausea, which immediately stopped the reaction, and he drifted off immediately for nearly half an hour due to the Benadryl.

The nurses were later able to finish the full dose of the third treatment, and Fred was able to go to the bathroom a couple times and walk. They said it was high unusual as most people handle the first part of the treatment badly but the end shots are fine—Fred had the strongest reaction that they had ever seen.

Fred Ho writes, "Tonight, the same drug continued via the portable pump hooked up by my visiting nurse Alison. Because it is at a much slower injection pace than the initial injection earlier today, and probably because my system is still filled with a lot of the drugs they used to counteract my earlier reaction, it went smoothly. I slept very, very well."

Note: Dr. Patel later told me that most likely I'm allergic to 5FU (one of the three chemo drugs in the FOLFOX regime) and that managing it would be done by a slow infusion rate as well as my taking Benadryl before the final infusion of that chemo drug.

DIARY 1: FRED HO PLAYS THE SAX AGAIN!

October 10, 2006

First, a very heartfelt and appreciative thank you to Mrs. Mary Sharp Cronson, visionary impresario and loving friend, who sent me $1,000 to help with the expenses in my battle against cancer. Mary is presenting the Guggenheim Museum Works and Process events November 5 and 6, 2006, at 7:30 PM, for which my music will be featured and at which I'll be in attendance and hope to see you all there.

Also, great news: though two weeks ago I tried to play the baritone sax and couldn't even manage to do thirty seconds, today, with the help and presence of singer-friend Jennifer Kidwell, I was able to play for thirty minutes! I could even reach into the fifth octave! While my dexterity is rusty and my embouchure weak, my diaphragm was good so my sound was strong. It made my day!

[Ann's note: In Jennifer's own words here's what she had to say, "I got to hang out with Fred today, and I wanted to let you know that Fred was able to play his sax for the first time in weeks! He sounded powerful and fabulous as usual. He played five songs for me at full volume, as well as scales and arpeggios. He said he's looking forward to practicing more. I'm looking forward to seeing his new pieces in performance in November."]

I have been losing a lot of weight. Since August 4, 2006, my colon cancer diagnosis, I've lost twenty-three pounds. My primary care physician is concerned that I'm losing too much weight too quickly and not getting enough calories, especially from protein. My appetite has been dampened by the chemo—from fatigue, nausea, and lack of taste buds. I also greatly miss Chinese food since the takeout restaurants in my neighborhood of Greenpoint all suck. I need someone educated in the good Lower Manhattan Chinese places who can do occasional take-out runs for me. I really miss *cha siu bao* (roast pork buns), something I've loved since I was a child and which I gave up for eleven years after I converted to Islam in the mid-1970s. I returned to eating pork by the late 1980s.

The experience with chemo has been unpredictable. Every day is uncertain. The first day home on Friday, October 6, 2006, was great. I woke up at sunrise and washed out my mouth (oral hygiene is crucially important to avoid infections through sores and gum lesions), copied out music parts, did paperwork, e-mails, made a large breakfast, walked a mile, a very overall active and full day. I went to bed just after 9:00 PM.

Day 2 was awful, filled with fatigue, nausea, no appetite, malaise. I could barely eat anything. The weather was cold and wet and dark, not helping. I baked a pie simply to turn on the oven and warm up my place and to try to eat something I would like, but I barely had appetite for the pie. The visiting nurse, Alison, came by at 8:15 PM to disconnect me from the portable chemo pump. I took medications before going to sleep.

Day 3, Sunday, was a good day. The sun was coming out. I could eat breakfast. My usual breakfast consists of fruit, high-quality bread with preserves, cottage cheese with flaxseed oil and fruit or fruit preserves (thanks to Jen Shyu for this dietary/nutritional method of cancer fighting), juice, and tea. I finished copying all my big band parts and felt satisfied in completing a project. Rick Ebihara from the fantastic Asian American performance theater group Slant visited and brought some Trader Joe's goodies. We talked for two hours—pure enjoyment.

Day 4, Monday, was a so-so day, with less appetite, fatigue. I didn't realize today was Columbus Day, a holiday, as I'm some what out of touch with the outside world. I just took it easy most of the day. Several old friends called during this holiday, and it was great chatting with them. The weather was warm and sunny, so I walked to the park and did long breathing exercises. I have begun to regularly do meditative breathing exercises. Later that afternoon I put on a CD of early blues music (copulatin' blues) and did tai chi movements to the music (a new Afro Asian activity!). I didn't go to bed until very late, after midnight, as I had a burst of energy and couldn't fall asleep and just got up and watched some movies. Earlier in the evening, my friends Gwen and Rick from the Bay Area called and recommended aloe vera and vitamin E oil to ease the irritation and pain of my scar and to ease the drying skin tissue and encrusted scabbing. I didn't have vitamin E oil around the home, but the aloe vera I did have worked great. Thank you!

Day 5, Tuesday, I woke up thinking I had slept until noon, but it was actually 9 AM, the latest I've slept since beginning chemo. The doorbell rang, which woke me up, and it was the mailman bringing a great care package from my warrior friends in Hawaii with two bottles of noni juice and two great CDs of Hawaiian music. They are mounting an e-mail campaign to get people to buy/download my music online to help me increase revenues. *Mahalo!*

During the rest of the morning, I began to read/research the question of "jazz" and the avant-garde and social change as part of a keynote speech I will give at the University of Kansas in late March 2007 after my chemo is done.

I met my agent/friend Joseph Yoon for lunch at the local Thai café. I was surprised how big of an appetite I had today, chowing down on a large plate of squid pad thai and a seafood basil dish.

I was feeling good, and as medical advice says, you don't lie down after one eats, so I walked around the neighborhood, visiting the local Salvation Army and found some wild clothes for the November 5 and 6 Guggenheim event, which if you all come, I'll surprise you and wear!

Daily, I drink a lot of water and juices and teas all the time to counter the effects of dehydration that are brought on by chemo and its side effects. I have stopped drinking cold beverages (nothing with ice) and have become a caffeine-free tea drinker.

I have been reading a lot of cancer literature to understand and anticipate what I will face.

Day 6 and 7: I meet a week prior to each chemo treatment visit with my oncologist, Dr. Patel, for blood work to monitor my red and white blood cell count to make sure they don't drop too much. My immune system is being destroyed by the chemo, and I must be carefully monitored. On Wednesday night, I came down with diarrhea—very rough. Took advanced Imodium.

WHAT CHANGES I'M GOING THROUGH

I can no longer be the type-A personality I have been, relying upon my stamina and willpower to go nonstop at high intensity. I have to take naps and breaks, as I'm physically unable to sustain an intense, concentrated, prolonged output. I am enjoying my breathing exercises, the immediate moments in conversation—without losing my ability, capacity, and desire to see a bigger picture and think with a radical imagination. I miss swimming, hand-to-hand combat workouts, performing, working hard, producing new projects; but I've come to gradually replace these things with reflection, breathing, patience, letting go, catching up with lots of old friends, and deepening my friendship and love with newer friends. I've enjoyed seeing my friends' children, some very new in this world, though I know now that I'm in chemo, I must hold off contact with the little people and their parents.

Something Mike, a new friend, told me that I'm beginning to see. He is a cancer survivor and said that cancer was a way for God to show him that he had still something to learn about life. While I'm a devout atheist, I do realize that this war is teaching me new things about myself, the world, the system we live in, and the philosophical conundrums of existence, life, reality, and love.

I have always been a fighter, but now I'm learning to fight on a cellular level. What I am coming to understand is that while I have never believed there to be a contradiction between materialism and spirituality, that if spirituality is to matter, then it must be materialist. It is the fight, rather than fatalism and faith, that matters. However, the fight is aided by faith, by the love and actions of both the individual and all around oneself. It is that basic interaction that makes our existence conditionally and ultimately social and interconnected and inextricable.

WHAT PEOPLE CAN SEND TO ME OR DO TO HELP ME:

1. No-Ad Aloe Vera moisturizing gel. Dry skin is a common side effect and gets worse with the dryness of winter.
2. Living plants that I can raise and increase the oxygen in my surroundings.
3. Take me on a trip to the botanical garden or greenhouse so I can breathe oxygen.
4. Go to NYC Chinatown and pick up some dim sum, some *cha siu bao*, and other things I like to eat and miss a lot.
5. I always need drivers.

6. Sharing ideas, talking, telling me stories, discussing future projects, etc. I love hearing about things in the outside world and among all of your lives.
7. Juices, a box/basket of fresh citrus fruits, fresh fruit preserves/jams, flaxseed oil, Trader Joe's green and very green juices, ginger-lemon-echinacea juice.
8. Biotene mouthwash, great stuff (nonalcohol) for oral hygiene.

I have enjoyed the many readings, books, CDs, movies/DVDs/videos people have sent. My ability to read for a length of time is still limited. I read a few pages, rest, read, or do something else.

Every day is uncertain and unpredictable. I have had to modify and change plans I begin with depending on my fatigue, energy, appetite, and strength. There are days I have tremendous energy and start at sunrise and go all day without a rest or a nap. Then there are days I can't seem to get any energy or feel awful. I just have to roll with it all.

DIARY 2: THE WARRIOR REFLECTS

October 13, 2006

I am daily convinced that fighting cancer is a war. It is a war fought on the medical/cellular level, it is a war fought on the social–economic-political level against the U.S. HMO system of profiteering off healthcare, and it is a war fought on the spiritual-physical-mental-manual level of yin-yang. I meet fellow warriors who are fighting cancer and veterans who have been through it and live to tell their stories and share their lessons and strategy and tactics. Some of these veterans are very militant, lecture and drill me with questions and "things to think about"; others simply listen. But in their hearts, they all come from a place, despite all of our differences, that we have been at war and know it.

I have chosen to share/discuss with all of you Warriors for Fred via the diary method, understanding that the greatest warriors, from Sun Tzu to swordsman Murasashi, to Bruce Lee, all wrote daily diaries because warfare against a most formidable enemy will be won ultimately on the *philosophical level* (combining physical tactics and strategy with a vision beyond simply defeating-controlling, but completely neutralizing the enemy by transforming the very conditions that produced the animosity, antagonism and conflict, and empowered the enemy to begin with). Many militarists and would-be conquerors have read Sun Tzu incorrectly and improperly, simply to gain tactics and strategy for accumulating victories. To paraphrase Sun Tzu, conquering is easy, transforming is hard. The militarists have stripped the ethical and purposive cornerstones from Sun Tzu. The warrior makes war *only* when attacked or facing grave threat, not for self-gain. The militarist employed to expand power and wealth and territory is simply a hired fighter, though perhaps very well trained and experienced. As I fight this war against cancer, I struggle to understand the true way of the warrior to fight for beauty, justice, health, equity, sustainability.

After a week of being off chemo, the days have become more normal with less bouts of nausea, fatigue, loss of appetite, coldness, malaise. I continue to practice my bari sax for at least thirty minutes every day. I am mostly practicing for sound and endurance, not technique. A new breakthrough: I am exercising again! (See more below.)

Shan Min Yu, a Chinese vocalist-actress I worked a lot with in the 1990s, came to visit (she now lives in Taiwan). She talked a lot about performances she'd like to do with me when I'm recovered, which uplifted my spirits a lot. I spend some of my time thinking about future projects, such as wanting to do a new opera based on Anthony and Cleopatra, a project with native Alaskan totem carver Stephen Jackson and dancer/choreographer Ashley Byler and writer-performer Keith Smith in Ketchitkan, Alaska, possibly summer of 2008, someday collaborating with native Hawaiian hula artists, an underwater ballet for synchronized swimmers called "Divas of the Deep," and many other ideas.

I am heartened by my friendship and professional collaboration with impresario Thaddeus Squire, founder-president of Peregrine Arts in Philadelphia. He is driving me to two chemo sessions and being my chemo companion so we can talk about our work together and come up with new ideas and plans. His paradigm in the performing arts, if you all allow me to share it with you, is so visionary: rather than the typical run-an-institution-put-on-a-season model, his approach is do-the-projects-you-want wherever/ whenever you want. It is driven by the value of the artist and the work and not by any institutional considerations whatsoever.

October 14, 2006

I had a breakthrough by beginning to exercise. I did thirty push-ups, fifteen behind-the-back chin-ups (though gingerly), three hundred horse stance waist bends, and three hundred circular waist sweeps.

I've decided the risk of going swimming in a public facility and exposure to germs is too great. I plan to continue daily walks but add in some new isometrics that I used to do back in the 1970s based on ideas developed by the late great Bruce Lee. I will push against walls, not to break or crack them, but to find a point of resistance/balance. I do circular waist bends and turns and light chin-ups. I will also do kung fu horse leg stances and stretches made famous by Wong Fei-hung, the inventor of tiger-crane and the greatest master of the no-shadow kick. Anyone who wants to work out with me, please come by! Strength isn't building big muscles/bulk, but strengthening tendons and ligaments.

Back in 1993 when I tore my Achilles' tendon and used natural, nonsurgery healing, once my cast was below the knee, out of my couch, I did all upper-body exercises for power and strength such as three hundred pushups, three hundred sit-ups, etc.

My strength and zone of struggle is no longer exterior, but interior; fighting cancer cells and maximizing flexibility; adaptability and resistance. Once I am in remission, I can rebuild the exterior, but without a cancer-free, highly oxygenated interior, the exterior won't matter. I see how the exercise industry is promoting all the wrong stuff (what else is new?). I am returning to a lot of ancient teachings and precepts of Asian martial arts to better understand the yin-yang (dialectical materialism) of righteous living. I shall periodically share what I'm learning in these diary entries. One kernel of insight from an early tai chi master: all solutions are found in nature. As our industrial society destroys and toxifies nature, we increasingly are eliminating what possible solutions we may have. There is a tipping point when quantity turns into qualitative change that is irreversible.

What all of you, my friends, have done, is help me rebuild and strengthen my inner being, to wage the war on a cellular level. This comes from the nutritious food, the non caffeinated teas, the plants and flowers that bring beauty and oxygen, the relief of stress by doing errands, cleaning my house, driving me to appointments, etc. That all of you have given and done. Of course, the prayers, chanting, well wishes are helpful too.

Once I have achieved this victory of strengthening my interior, rebuilding the exterior is simple and easy. For example, once my diaphragm healed, I can now play the sax. Technique and embouchure will be easy to regain. And perhaps the new breathing exercises, slower counter/non Alpha personality modalities will do more to strengthen the diaphragm and hence improve my playing in all of this.

Once I have truly won the war (I'll know in about ten years), I will have achieved two transformations: the spirit/soul is empowered to fight at the cellular level, and the exterior will not be what it was ten years ago when the tumor first developed (I plan to be living differently, have different behavioral practices, and eliminate my exposure to toxicity (social, psychological, personal/people, and environmental). If I have to, I am prepared to sell everything and move far away from industrial society. I invite any and all who want to join me.

I went to bed at 9:00 PM.

October 15, 2006

Woke up at 6:00 AM and briskly walked to McCarren Park half a mile away to do a workout so that I am not exposed to the sunshine (my skin cells have died, and new skin is slowly growing, but it is like virgin baby skin and burns easily). Improved my push-ups to forty-five today.

My old friend Jamala and her seventy-five-year-old mother Lollie came into town to celebrate their birthdays to see the Broadway show *The Color Purple* and trekked out to see me this morning.

At 11:00 AM, Aib Gomez-Delgado, Taylor Ho Bynum, Ayesha, and I piled into Taylor's small car and went to NYC Chinatown so I could "educate" them in the best Chinese restaurants to get take outs I like. I showed them where to get *cha siu bao* (roast pork buns, both steamed and baked), great noodle joints, great vegetarian and seafood places, and how to order. I've always maintained that with a great Chinatown, no one really needs to cook (especially during hot summer months); they just need to know where to go and what to order. Now I have my fix for Chinese food solved! Anyone else who wants to be educated, just call and come by!

Breathing long, deep, slow breaths is helping many things. Besides restful and calming, it is actually helping my sinuses. After two surgeries in 2002 and 2004 respectively for sleep apnea and nonmalignant polyp growth inside my nose and throat, I have a lot of scar tissue. Some of you may recall that I was in constant irritation with constant postnasal drip. Well, I seem to have "managed" (a corporate term doctors are using/saying when they can't "solve" something and want to get you to adjust and accommodate to something you shouldn't have to) to relieve a lot of this problem not through any chemical sprays but simply "exercising" my nose/breath regularly, possibly helping to heal the bad scar issue inside my nose. That and the fact I've lost a lot of weight helps. The other benefit is that I am *listening* more to my breath. It tells me how I'm doing.

I cook for myself, but I really enjoy both the food and the company that people bring when they visit. I learn a lot about people through their foods and what they make. Yumi Kurosawa, *koto* musician, makes terrific Japanese tofu, seaweed, and chicken meatball soup spiced with shredded ginger and soy sauce. Anything Gladys Serrano, arts administrator, touches seems to turn out delicious. Her Puerto Rican rice and beans and seafood Creole casserole were wiped out by me. Paget Walker's turkey pot pie, eaten soon after I got out of surgery, was devoured without a scrap left. Maori visual artist DM Wilding prepared a banquet meal that was expansive and scrumptious. Ayesha made an out-of-this-world Indian chicken biryani with yogurt and cucumber (I never ate yogurt until now!). All the dishes everyone made and brought were filled with their spirit of caring and love. As Magdalena said, "You can taste the love!"

I realize that Western medicine is based on *cut-burn-poison* while Chinese medicine is based on food and largely preventative. While I have to be very careful with the interaction of herbs and homeopathic approaches with the highly toxic chemotherapy, I will employ a Chinese approach to healing with food, breathing, exercise and *philosophical contemplation* (which I prefer *over* the highly Western-commercialized fad of "meditation") since I believe one heals/changes oneself through changing the world/society rather than apolitical solipsism. I listen to my breath and to the music of others, to the breath of many others.

Part of my healing is healing old issues or rifts with longtime friends. People I've known since my youth have been calling and e-mailing. We have "cleared the air," another important part of breathing!

October 16–18, 2006

I've increased my push-ups to seventy-five a day.

The days get better and better farther from the chemo and then back to the chemo every two weeks. I get up around sunrise and exercise in the park, walk a mile every day at least, answer mail and e-mail, and start to work on new projects. Daily I practice the sax for at least forty-five minutes or more. Laura Whitehorn and Idell Conaway have been kind and generous in sending me some financial assistance.

I learned that the poet-writer Chiori Santiago has breast cancer. I sent her some money, some music, some books, and pictures. I don't know her personally, but was told about her war from an old friend-comrade-writer Genny Lim (who got a book published recently by the Ministry of Culture in Venezuela, where she was bestowed national honors by President Chavez, after fifty years of struggling with very little recognition or rewards here in her home country, the United States. Viva Hugo Chavez!).

I continue to have a good appetite and am eating a lot of pasta and seafood and meatballs to put on more weight. I've returned to drinking no-fat organic cow's milk made by Eco-Dairy. I had given up eating morning cereal forty years ago, but now I have a high-fructose corn-syrup-*free* cereal (whole grains and whole wheat) with fruit (bananas, blackberries, apples, etc.) or I have an Asian breakfast of noodles, meat, and veggies. All this with a multivitamin and plenty of different juices and, of course, *tea*.

October 19, 2006: second chemo out
of twelve (ten more to go!)

Not to worry, today's second out of twelve chemo treatments had no drama like the first one. The nurse/doctors learned from what happened and drugged me first and then did the infusion slower than before. I got to the hospital at 8:30 AM to do my blood tests, and my blood count numbers were good.

At 10:30 AM after the blood results came back and the premeds were done, they began the chemo (three drugs, two first, then the 5FU last). The last injection began around 1:45 PM. Because they gave me Benadryl first, I fell asleep quickly and slept for almost two hours. I only woke up to go pee and noticed how late it was. Thaddeus, who drove me and was my chemo companion, also fell asleep. He said watching me sleep made him sleepy!

But there was no reaction to the infusion this time.

The visiting nurse Alison hooked me up around 7:00 PM tonight. She'll call me tomorrow to see how I'm doing and return Saturday at 8:00 PM after forty-nine hours to disconnect me.

She said that probably last time, I did too much on the Friday so that's maybe why on Saturday I was feeling awful. She said that the two days I'm on the portable pump I shouldn't go out, should just take it easy. And then late in the day on Saturday, see people and do things as the chemo is running out. I'll take her advice.

Luckily, I've stocked up on enough food and supplies to last two to three days without going out.

So what I'll do on day 1 to 3 of chemo is really just rest, no workouts, no practicing, no running around, and no visitors (sorry). That might help make my chemo trip smoother.

DIARY 3: BED AND BENADRYL

October 20, 2006

The third week has been one of constant fatigue, long hours of sleep, and general inactivity, a marked contrast from the first two weeks with volatility, ups and downs, and an ascending improvement moving further from the chemo treatment cycle. This week I had a marked drop in activity, barely able to exercise or play the sax. The one constant I am able to sustain is deep breathing and to listen very closely to what my breath tells me.

Love and thanks to Jayne Cortez for advancing me $300 for our next music-poetry project.

Day 2 of chemo, at home on the portable chemo pump. Last night, I couldn't sleep. Possibly from the steroids I was pumped with during the hospital treatment in combination with having napped for two hours from the Benadryl. I didn't fall asleep until after 5:00 Am and woke up today just before 11:00 AM. I'm taking the advice of Nurse Alison and taking it easy. Watched on DVD *X-Men 3: The Last Stand*. I get all choked up from good superhero comic book movies.

Michi Kanno set me some organic tea, two meditational chanting CDs, and Egyptian skin cream to help with my scar and skin dryness. Thank you, Michi.

Friends from the Civitella Raineri Foundation sent me a year long membership to the Brooklyn Botanical Garden. Thank you so much for responding to this specific request that will help oxygenate me.

So for days 1–3 of chemo, I will not exercise or practice the sax or go outside unless I absolutely have to. I will go out for walks daily, but not push it with multiple errands, etc. As improvement happens from days 4 to 14, I will gradually step up the activities as normalcy returns. I am still learning what patterns, if any, will manifest for the next five and a half months longer of chemo.

Dehydration is a constant threat. The water bottle given to me by Marsha Lawson last Christmas has been very useful as frequently during my sleep I must take swigs from it to stay hydrated. Fluids are a big part of my daily intake, from teas to water to all kinds of juices (noni, pomegranate, green magma superfood combinations, fruit shakes, and my favorite Trader Joe's lemon-ginger-echinecea). I always welcome a gift of a gallon of bottled water or any kind of juice.

I spend a good portion of my day replying to letters and e-mails. I have vowed to answer every single correspondence. My heart is touched by the many who have reached out.

I took Benadryl to help me fall asleep.

October 21, 2006, Day 3 of Chemo

It seems day 3 (Saturday) of chemo is the worst. I woke up around 11:00 AM (that Benadryl is powerful stuff). Very groggy, slight nausea. Tightening of my rear jaw (which the hospital staff warned might be a side effect). Some chills but not as bad as the first Saturday after chemo.

I just didn't have the energy to read books or do much other than watch some movies, read some e-mails, and just rest. Had barely any appetite and had to force myself to eat.

I did go out for a short walk to the local Saturday farmers' market to pick up some vegetables.

Alison, the visiting nurse, came by in the evening to disconnect my chemo. She noticed that I had a red rash on my chest, the same symptom that happened in the hospital two weeks ago.

Since I can't wash when I have the chemo infusions, I finally took a shower tonight and went to bed.

October 22, 2006

I didn't use Benadryl last night, but I was so exhausted that I slept to 10:00 AM this morning. Every one and a half to two hours while in bed at night I have to get up and hydrate. Dehydration is a constant threat. Because I'm drinking a lot of liquids, I have to pee constantly as well. The ability to sleep steadily through the night isn't possible. The chemo has affected the scar healing on my stomach, slowing it down. I also have constant irritation from the scar tissue. A blanket touching my stomach can be very irritating. I sometimes put a plastic bucket on top of my stomach to hold the blanket from touching my skin.

For most of today, I was feeling very tired, low energy. I also was very clumsy in the morning, dropping things. I hope this isn't the side effect of peripheral neuropathy (loss of dexterity and pain in outer limbs). I'll have to see how my sax playing goes the next few days.

The candles that people have sent I have cautiously begun to use in a limited aroma therapy. I am still cautious about burning too much as I have to do more research on the relationship of inhalation of anything burning as a carcinogen. But the scent seems to have a relaxing effect on me.

Marty Khan sent me an e-mail about how the music of John Coltrane (especially the works of "A Love Supreme," "Spiritual," etc.) has helped him lower his blood pressure. I too have found this effect with Trane's music but also a lot of preindustrial primal music (e.g., Kim Tinsley sent two CDs of Gnawa ritual trance and possession music). I am convinced that the vibrations of acoustic music (best *live*), particularly the more shamanistic, the greater the healing power. When recovering from surgery, the trancelike inducement of this music helped me to zone out the TV sets, the inane conversations, etc., bombarding our aural senses. It also helped me to dance (lying on my back!), to move my limbs and pelvis, rotate my ankles and wrists.

October 23, 2006

I couldn't sleep very well again last night. Woke up at 5:00 AM and couldn't fall back asleep. Feeling very listless, tired, no energy, but a lot less nausea, which is good. I practiced the sax today for about thirty minutes. No problems there. Not having much appetite. Have to force myself to eat.

John Duffy was visiting from Maine and came by to see me. It's good to see the hero of American new music, the founder of Meet the Composer. He championed me at a time when no one would.

In the evening, Joseph Franklin and Laurel Wycoff called. They live in Albuquerque. Laurel works for the State government delivering food to the needy. She warned me about the MLM (multilevel marketing, a.k.a. pyramid) schemes related to noni, pomegranate, and mangosteen juices. Apparently back in 1993, conservative Utah Senator Orrin Hatch prevented the FDA from medically evaluating all so-called homeopathic remedies as many are manufactured and distributed in Utah. The alternative medicine lobby didn't want its products to be scientifically tested and possibly exposed. Currently, you read the labeling, and there are lots of praises and testimonies of curative claims (e.g., "Helps support immune system") with the provision "This statement has not been evaluated by the FDA. This product is not intended to diagnose, treat, cure or prevent any disease."

I believe, however, there are antioxidant benefits to these juices, but certainly as these juices become trendier, not justifying the price.

October 24, 2006

This week has had a lot more side effects. Today I woke up at 5:00 AM and went to the park and worked out but could only do two-thirds of what had become an almost-normal workout last week. I returned home and made breakfast and then fell asleep again and slept for most of the day. I am filled with anemia. Last Saturday, I had a red chest while the portable chemo was being infused. During the mornings I experienced tightness of my jaw. Along with this, in the mornings I had some slight headaches.

Today I couldn't do much at all except sleep and make myself dinner. In the middle of the night, I experienced a very painful stiffening of all my joints (elbows, knees). It was hard to walk at night to the bathroom.

October 25, 2006

Again, I slept most of the day except for making myself breakfast, lunch, and a very light dinner; answering e-mails; checking the mailbox. I did do some light reading. Couldn't even watch TV or a movie.

Wednesdays after chemo treatments seem to be the diarrhea day.

I have to really just roll with everything. Be willing to revise according to what my body tells me.

Marina Celander came to visit bringing a beautiful plant. Plants are beginning to fill my apartment.

October 26, 2006

Plants keep multiplying in my small apartment, especially herbal ones such as rosemary, basil, oregano, along with dandelions and a bamboo tree that Ruth Margraff brought over with a dragon curled around the pot.

I had to wait more than two hours in the wait room for my bimonthly appointment with my oncologist Dr. Patel. While waiting, I read that in 1996 the American Cancer Society stated that a million and a half people were diagnosed with some kind of cancer. No wonder the oncology rooms and doctors are so swamped.

Good news: all my blood counts were strong. Red blood cells (which transmit oxygen and fight anemia), white blood cells (which are your immune system and fight infections), and platelets (which support blood clotting and prevent you from bleeding to death) are all very good. I have also gained weight, and my blood pressure has increased to 150/92. There are several possible factors for this: anxiety from the chemo therapy, since I drink a lot of juice, teas, etc., the increased potassium and sodium.

As far as jaw tightening and joint pain side effects, Dr. Patel prescribed increased calcium and magnesium, as needed.

Prof. Peter Rachleff and Prof. Beth Cleary of Macalester College in St. Paul, Minnesota, visited today. Beth was so terrific in running around doing errands for me like getting my eyeglasses repaired, etc. Thank you for visiting!

Thanks to my buddy Arthur Song who has been staying in NYC as often as he can (he lives in Amsterdam, the Netherlands) to help me. He bought a case of fifteen bottles of Biotene mouthwash today—that should last a year!

October 27, 2006

A really good night's sleep, woke up at 7:30 AM as the sun rose. Today feels like it will be a good day. More to come in the next war diary.

DIARY 4: SHOULDER TO SHOULDER

*Week 4: Chemo Treatment Number 3 (Nine More to Go)**
October 30 to November 10, 2006

*Former political prisoner Laura Whitehorn remarked how counting down the chemo treatments is like when prisoners tick off the days they have left on their sentence!

In the second chemo cycle, days 1 to 10 were filled with a lot of fatigue and long hours of sleep. Finally, on day 11 (Sunday, October 29), I woke up feeling I had slept enough and that the remaining days in this cycle were going to be better ("better" meaning able to go a whole day without sleeping, able to exercise, enjoy eating, and actually be able to taste and savor food, play the sax, read, and "work" on something, in other words, having a day that feels somewhat normal with no side effects).

This latest third chemo cycle, days 1 to 7 were tiring but not as intense fatigue as the last cycle. While I had to take naps, rest, and take it easy (and wasn't able to exercise), I didn't find myself constantly facing a bone-tired sleepiness. Some patterns are emerging:

> Day 1 treatment infusion in the hospital, the Benadryl makes me want to sleep as soon as I return home. Day 2 is not a bad day, and I can manage some light activity. Day 3, the final day on the portable chemo pump at home is usually the worst with nausea and exhaustion, peripheral neuropathy. Days 4–5 are better, but I use them to simply rest and overcome the three prior days of chemo infusion. Days 6–7 improve, though day 7 (Wednesday) have usually had diarrhea by the evening. The days I look forward to resuming some normalcy are days 8 to 14.

Special thanks and love to John Duffy for his care package of blueberry and pomegranate juices, a CD of his wonderful music, and his beautiful hand-drawn get-well card.

Also to Ms. Baraka Sele for her loving gift of $100.

To Peggy Choy for traveling from Madison, Wisconsin, to visit me and bringing some green magma powder to increase my chlorophyll intake, for bringing a Native American medicine wheel and for giving me a reiki energy treatment.

And to all the warriors and friends who came to the November 5 and 6 shows at the Guggenheim Musuem, including (and please forgive me if I forgot anyone) the following: Magdalena Gómez, Jim Lescault, Laura Whitehorn, Ann T. Greene and Mark O'Ferrall (and for driving me on Sunday to the event), Paget Walker, Peggy Choy, Jesse Wardlow (visiting from Chicago), Jennifer Kidwell, Marina Celander, Akiko Hiroshima, Sonoko Kawahara, Daystarr and Evergreen, Jayne Cortez and Mel Edwards, Linda Kwon (visiting from Seoul, Korea), Tom Buckner, Paola Prestini, Cia Toscanni (from ASCAP), Ashley Byler and Stephen Jackson, Dawn Akemi Saito, Jeff Janisheski, Daria Fain and Robert Kocik, Jen Shyu, Anka Lupes (thank you for giving me a plant!), DM Wilding, Deb Gilbert and Scott Kegelsmann, and to Ruth Margraff for driving me on Monday night!

Of course, to Howard Stokar and Mary Sharp Cronson for inviting me to be one of the guest composers for a terrific celebration of the poetry of James Tate. And to Ray Franks on baritone sax and the incredible vocal talents of Haleh Abghari! You two rock!

Do I have keloids? One of the oncologists at my weekly visit remarked that *keloids* had formed from my stomach scar. Keloids, as I have researched, are most common to women and people of African descent. Some East Asian Indians and Chinese get them. They are bumpy ridges, looking like armadillo armor or Klingon forehead bumps (for you *Star Trek* fans). They aren't harmful, but are considered "unsightly." First discovered in Ancient Egypt around 1400 BCE, they were self-inflicted as "warrior scarification" by certain African peoples as signification of toughness and bravery.

But in my visit to my surgeon, Dr. Berman, he dismissed this diagnosis of keloids and said this was simply normal process of scar healing.

Describing how chemo feels. I have been searching for a way to describe, both for myself and to all of you, what it feels like to be going through chemotherapy. Chemotherapy is the use of highly powerful, toxic drugs that kill all new cell growth (both the bad cancer cells which are more active and multiply faster than good, healthy cells). When the drugs are being injected into me (days 1–3 of the chemo cycle), I feel dry, brittle, like my very life essence is being drained. The best short description is that I feel "dried out." Like plants leaves when they dry out, getting brittle, my energy zapped away. I notice on my bedsheets that dead skin sheds more at the beginning of the chemo cycle. I am constantly thirsty. I eat, but there is no joy, no sense of being refueled with new energy. My skin feels prickly, parched. On bad days, I am nauseous, very exhausted. When exposed to cold, my fingers and hands get tingly and numb (a side effect called peripheral neuropathy). This is easily remedied by either putting on gloves or warming my body by leaving the cold. Usually one day out of the fourteen I have diarrhea. The diarrhea either runs its course in three toilet goings, or I use advanced Immodium, which usually fixes it. Of the fourteen days in between my chemo treatments, so far, if one week is side effect free, then I'm doing well.

Laryngeal spasms. This is a troubling side effect of the particular chemo I am getting. It is triggered by cold air (either breathing it in say when I open the freezer, or from being outside in cold weather). The cold triggers constriction of the throat and can lead to major breathing difficulties. To prevent this, I need to be very careful and wear a scarf in cold weather and avoid breathing cold air.

Dietary experiment and analysis. I have been searching for the best and most effective dietary approach to fighting the effects of chemo and to enhance my overall anticancer regimen. I find that what works best so far is a very diverse meal and constant variety. While plenty of water is very important, different kinds of teas and juices and other drinks (shakes without ice) are helpful. Combining a variety of carbo sources (rice, whole-grain breads, oatmeal, cereals, etc.), a variety of protein (beef, pork, chicken, fish, seafood, beans–legumes), plenty of fresh raw and cooked vegetables, different fruits, and different cultural cuisines (Mediterranean, south and east Asian) seem to work best. I have eliminated most cheese (except for grated on pasta), creams, eggs (except when cooked in Asian dishes), reduced added salt, try to avoid all preservatives, and absolutely eliminated trans fats and hydrogenated oils. The elimination of most processed foods and the increase of raw foods (including raw fish—sushi and sashimi) seems to give me the best energy. I rarely eat any dessert now. I have also eliminated most Latin American and Caribbean foods, which I used to like and eat a lot of. The high-fat and fried-oil content seems to have an energy-depleting effect on me.

The American Cancer Society, the U.S. mainstream cancer organization, advocates the following dietary approach to cancer resistance: limit red meats and animal fats; stop eating deep-fried foods, reduced refined and processed foods; eliminate alcohol consumption and certainly cigarette smoking, etc. While not saying that these things "cause" cancer (except constant cigarette smoking), the ACS warns of "evidence to suggest" that barbequed and smoked-cooked foods (including broiled fish—anything cooked at high temperatures) has been linked to increases in cancer risk.

Cancer-fighting/reducing risk foods include raw fruits and vegetables and high antioxidant sources from juices, whole grains, oats, and many other high-fiber sources.

The area of alternative, complementary, and integrative medical approaches are under-researched by mainstream cancer research and medical institutions.

Lessons from postsurgery recovery. I received a thank-you card from Nurse Ashlyn Hyacinthe saying that my letter of commendation to her bosses at the North Shore Long Island Jewish Hospital about her excellent care giving while I was recovering from surgery truly helped her career. Receiving her card triggered my memories about some very important lessons I learned from postsurgery recovery in the hospital.

Once you leave the operating table and are wheeled into the recovery ward, healing and recovery is *all on you, the patient.* The doctors visit once a day to make sure nothing is seriously awry. The nurses check on your vitals and make sure none of your numbers are not where they shouldn't be. If you are lucky and have caring, knowledgeable and helpful nurses, and patient care advocates (the nurses' assistants, the people who change your sheets, wash you, bring you water, your meals, etc.), as I for the most part did (though there were two bad exceptions, whom I reported and requested be fired), they are your allies and in-hospital support system. Your friends and family who visit are your out-of-hospital allies who advocate for you. The more proactive and greater presence they exert, the more "notice" the hospital staff is put on to watch out for you and to be as professional as they can. I was lucky to have such great tactful and tough enforcers as Jennifer Feil and Magdalena Gómez who made sure *all* the hospital staff knew about me. They demanded that one nurse, who was incompetent and negligent, be not allowed to administer to me.

Your worst problem is the other patients. So many give up, are despondent, neglected without visitors who care or love them, who think that they needn't do anything in terms of their own self-recovery, and that it's the doctors' job to fix them. They just watch TV all day and night at full volume or have idiotic conversations on the telephone. They disturb your peace, rest, and ability to heal. They can be obnoxious, inconsiderate, and a pain in the ass. They won't even take the simplest steps toward their own recovery and create a very depressing psychological environment.

As soon as you can, and the nurses will tell you when you can, usually within twenty-four hours after surgery, you *must* get out of bed and walk. Movement is the best thing for you. Lying in bed on your back all the time is the worst thing. Daily movement, intellectual stimulation, peace of mind, constant hydration, and having a positive, self-empowered attitude are keys to a thorough and quicker recovery. A big part of *healing* is psycho-spiritual. Feeling good about oneself, of noticing recovery and improvement, of being confident that you can return to your home and normal activity are all things that *only you* can do for yourself.

FIGHTING THE CANCER WAR ON MULTIPLE FRONTS

There is no one primary cause of cancer. Factors include genetics (since cancer is a mutation of normal, healthy genes, bombarded by cancer-favorable environmental stimuli and certain genetic-encoded predisposition), exposure to carcinogens, and specific and general environmental toxicity (radiation from the sun, exacerbated by the shredding of the earth's ozone; intensified electromagnetic radiation; accumulation of pesticides and contaminants in our food and water sources; growth-inducing hormones and stimulants in our food supply; the increase in toxins from overall pollution and overabundance in our foods and pharmaceutical ingestion; etc.).

Since cancer has a multiplicity of causal factors, it is logical to assume that the war against cancer requires a multiplicity of fronts to fight on, including the medical, nutritional, spiritual, and behavioral. The greatest benefit that all of you have given to me is motivational and inspirational through your love, friendship, caring, support, and direct assistance. I feel most invigorated and alive when people visit and have discussions with me. Colleagues are visiting and meeting with me, planning and preparing new projects. The offers to help find me gigs after my chemo, whether they be performances, speaking engagements, presenting papers at conferences, etc., keep me active and engaged.

While some days I may not feel well to see people or socialize, there are other days when I'm hungry for companionship and hanging out. While I have decided to not go out to public events of any kind to minimize my risk to germs and illnesses, I enjoy and crave people coming over and giving me their reviews, sharing me new music and reading materials, and conversing on all topics.

Not once through this war have I felt defeat, depression, or despondency. Frustration, yes, mostly from the abysmal medical system we have in the United States. Fear, yes, from heavy decisions that need to be made. Fatigue, yes, from the powerful chemo drugs. But I have never felt alone, isolated, or at a loss as to who to call on for help and support. I feel all of you are shoulder to shoulder with me in this war. And each of you brings their own special approaches and contributions to the fight, creating a diversity and multiplicity of fighting factors that I know, combined and united, will make this fight victorious!

DIARY 5: NO SORBET, NO PEACE

Week 5, Chemo Session Number 4 (Eight More to Go!)
November 11, 2006

Good news! The American Composers Orchestra has commissioned me to compose a twelve- to fifteen-minute concerto for baritone saxophone and chamber orchestra work to premiere February 8, 2008, at Carnegie Hall and also possibly in Philadelphia. Thanks to Derek Bermel, composer-in-residence at the ACO and friend and fellow warrior, for championing me.

Thank you to Samantha Smart and her kids for sending two big boxes of organic Italian orange juice bottles and assorted organic fruits.

And thanks to my literary agent Frances Goldin for her financial gift and thoughtful letter. She continues to be an extraordinary activist for low-income housing, for Mumia Abu-Jamal's freedom, and for being a steadfast anti-imperialist.

November 12, 2006

David Bindman picked me up to have a delicious Chinese brunch. We were joined by Kim Tinsley who, after eating, drove myself and her to Brooklyn to pick up Marina Celander, and the three of us went to the Brooklyn Botanical Garden (a year membership courtesy of the Civitella Raineri Foundation folks) to breathe oxygen all afternoon. Marina and Kim got me more plants for my apartment.

I am slowly excising red meat. Growing evidence suggest a higher risk for most cancers from eating red meat five times a week. I'm also cutting out all nonhome-cooked Latino food: too much oil, fat, salt. I used to love pernil, but I can feel it is tumor-feeding food. Certainly all deep-fried foods are gone. The best diet is macrobiotic and Japanese (miso soup is very good with fermented soy paste), though to two three decades ago, there was much hostility from the American Medical Association toward the advocates of this dietary regimen (and hostility and skepticism to most alterative approaches). The AMA seems to be slightly easing up as a more red-meat and high-fat and -sodium diet seems to be far more at risk to all kinds of cancers and other ailments than the vegetarian-prone dietary regimens. Ah, the politics of capitalism—the state—and the medical industry.

November 13–14, 2006

These were very good days. Even though the weather wasn't too good outside, I was able to practice the sax, get work done, begin planning the concerto commission, think about future projects and ideas, get a lot of reading and studying done. But over the weekend, I noticed my refrigerator wasn't staying cold and the frozen food was melting. I had to throw out all my ice cream and sorbet. Get rid of a lot of the frozen food and some perishables that rotted in my refrigerator including a head of broccoli, seafood, leftovers, a jar of mayo, a half-finished half gallon of fresh-squeezed carrot juice, etc. I called the repair service on Monday, who promised a repair person on Tuesday, who never showed, and the company wasted my whole day waiting for them ("wasted" because I couldn't go outside and do anything as I had to stay at home for their arrival, but nonetheless, I read and did other things).

Also, my toaster oven died. I hope to buy a good secondhand one from my local church tag sale, if it hasn't been sold yet.

And my receiver amp that I had repaired seems to not have been repaired. There's bleeding from the radio into the phono right speaker output, which interferes in my listening to phono LPs. Most of my music is LP vinyl. So much of the music I truly love will never be reissued as CDs because they never sold well (which is why I love them: great music/art doesn't often see commercial success unless much later, usually after the artists are dead, they become hot and trendy).

Even pop music that once did well but somehow falls through the cracks of corporate machinery, like the albums made by the jazz-rock band led by trumpeter Bill Chase, weren't reissued as CDs in the United States. I listen to pre-1980s American pop music and find it musically so much better than the 1980s-onward pop music with the exception of some early hip-hop like NWA Posse or Public Enemy. The

Chase 3 CDs have marvelously complex and brilliant four-trumpet arrangements and extraordinary altissimo work. The era of great lead trumpeters like Bill Chase, Maynard Ferguson, Cat Anderson, Doc Severinson, Snooky Young, Jon Faddis, players who night after night can hit double-high Cs and above to double-high Fs and Gs and even triple-high Cs, is over. We are in the Wynton Marsalis–Dave Douglas era, and the disappearance of steady Big Bands, has led to a generation of trumpet players unable and unfamiliar with the role of lead trumpeting playing. Great soloists like Dizzy Gillespie led big bands for many years and could embrace both the lower-range soloist and the high-range lead trumpet roles interchangeably. That's because a soloist, usually first, had to do a major stint in the big bands before becoming leader soloists. Wynton and Dave Douglas never paid their dues in the big band ranks.

To be a baritone saxophonist, of any era, with possibly the exception of Gerry Mulligan, you couldn't help but do the big bands as few small bands employed baritonists as frontline horn players. I think Mulligan had great lyrical solo ideas, but never the big, huge sound that must go with playing the baritone sax. That sound can only be developed when you have to anchor a seventeen-piece big band night after night. I learned that and acquired my sound from the years I spent in Charlie Persip's Superband, the subbing I did for the Gil Evans big band and Archie Shepp's Attica Blues Big Band. And from the years of playing the Basie, Thad Jones, Ellington big band charts.

November 15, 2006

Usually, the last day of my chemo cycle is the best. But today I woke up early, around 7:00 AM and felt very tired. I spent the whole morning fighting, which probably explains why by 2:00 PM I was completely exhausted and had to take a three-hour nap.

I was fighting the service contractor for Frigidaire since my refrigerator-freezer broke down this past weekend, and the company was supposed to send on a repair person on Tuesday, but that person never showed. Rather than call me and tell me the repair person didn't show up for work, they wasted my whole day waiting. They said they'd send him on Friday.

Then I had to fight with the Long Island Jewish Medical Center. I called and faxed both Dr. Patel, my oncologist, his research, nursing, and administrative staff, along with the quality management person (they don't have a "patient advocate," meaning someone whose job is the advocate for the patients' rights, rather someone who oversees the job performance of their staff). I was frustrated that the LIJMC and my HMO, Health Plus, have not straightened the misclassification of the LIJMC oncologists as "internists" (internal medicine physicians), which has obstructed my getting my primary care physician, Dr. Chen, and his clinic staff from getting the proper referrals *required* to authorize payments for my chemo and other doctor's visits. The matter got a bit testy and adversarial. Finally, Dale Janson, a research associate involved in my clinical trial and who has consistently tried to be helpful even though this is not his area of expertise, got on the phone both with the LIJMC provider relations department (who deal with the HMOs) and someone over at Health Plus to straighten this out. Hopefully, soon, this will be resolved. But after our initial phone call, which ended badly, we had agreed I would leave the clinical trial and suspend my treatments since I couldn't be assured that these costs would be covered by Health Plus, either future or even retroactively.

I then spent a lot of time trying to comb through the Health Plus directory and find a new oncologist. I called my sister, Florence Houn, who works for the cancer drugs section of the FDA in DC to help, and she got on her database to scrutinize the various Health Plus–provider oncologists for their qualifications in colorectal cancer.

After I got off the phone with Florence, Dale Janson called to say he feels confident that this will be worked out properly and asked me to reconsider. We both agreed that it would be best for me to continue my treatments and visits to the LIJMC.

I tried to cobble together a lunch to eat since I had to throw away a lot of my food. And then I went to sleep.

At 7:00 PM the director Jeff Janesheski came over to discuss directing a reading of the text-script for a new work, *Dragon vs. Eagle*, that Ruth Margraff and I are cowriting, which will take place January 20 and 21, 2006, at the Apollo Theater Salon (black box second floor). I was very tired, but we had a very good meeting. As soon as Jeff left, I went to bed, exhausted.

Access-A-Ride arrived five minutes early, but I was prepared having gone to meet them outside my apartment building ten minutes before the scheduled 6:41 AM pick up time. This is a good sign. I arrived one hour early for my 8:00 AM appointment. Luckily the ambulatory chemotherapy treatment center was open, and I simply sat and read the newspaper and the books I brought with me.

The chemotherapy went smoothly. First, the two-hour infusion of Leucovorin and Oxaliplatin. Then the dread last push of 5FU (*fluorouracil,* which has triggered reactions from me. This time they gave me 100 mg of Benadryl (double the usual 50 mg dosage). Wow, was I knocked out. I set my watch alarm for 2:25 PM so I wouldn't oversleep and meet Jon Ogilvy for my ride home. When I woke up, I was extremely drowsy and groggy. I could walk and go to the bathroom. Jon was so great to be there one hour ahead of the scheduled pickup time. I just felt bad I was barely able to stay awake in the car and was pretty lousy company for him. Thank you, Jon!

I got home and went to bed immediately. Alison, the visiting nurse, called me and said she'd be over soon and arrived at 7:00 PM to hook me up to the portable chemo (continuation of the 5FU infusion). I was able to make a light dinner and watched TV for an hour and then went back to bed. I didn't take any Benadryl, but the large dosage I got from hospital was still lingering, so I fell asleep easily. I woke up constantly from the need to drink water, to pee, and from the series of dreams I was having.

Here is one funny and strange dream:

I had just attended in the near future a concert at the Brooklyn Academy of Music by the Ojays. After the concert, there was an audience discussion led by BAM executive producer Joe Melillo. To get discussion flowing, he asked people he saw questions. He came to me and, knowing me well from the many shows I've done at BAM, asked me, "Fred, could you discuss the connections between black popular music of the 1970s and interest in Asian martial arts among black youth in particular during that period?"

Here is what I expounded:

Joe, the 1970s was an apex internationally and domestically of Third World peoples' national liberation struggles. Internationally, the peoples of Asia, Africa, and the Americas (Central, South and even oppressed nationalities in the United States and Canada) were kicking the ass of the U.S. government and military, with the leading example being the Vietnamese (both in the so-called North and South). Domestically, the Black Panthers served that leadership, along with the movements of Chicanos, Puertoriquenos, Asian/ Pacific Islander peoples and the American Indian Movement. Popular culture of that era couldn't help but express the era. The martial arts movies of Asia represented to black youth the desire to see people in the Third World kicking the white man's ass, or politically, kicking the butt of U.S. imperialism.

The audience was silent and then roared with applause and support. Joe said, "Thank you, Fred. We can always count on you for your provocative and invigorating comments."

Then in another dream I had, I commented to an audience interested in "jazz and the avant-garde": "The best of the jazz tradition celebrates and embraces individuality, which isn't the same as individualism. I oppose individualism, while I support individuality. Individualism is "Me! Me! Me!" Individuality is "I." "Me" is a possessive, therefore acquisitive, and as the "me, me, me, me, me, etc." mantra conveys, a mounting, incessant accumulative impetus. "I" is a singular subject, therefore an identity. (e.g., "I want it.") Ponder the distinctive difference between the proposition, "Give it to me!" versus "I want it!"

November 17, 2006: Day 2 of Chemo Cycle Number 4

I woke up at 4:00 AM and couldn't fall back asleep, so I proceeded to check e-mails and continue my Web research on cancer. I have found that the trace mineral selenium has shown promise as a disease-fighting enhancement in supporting antioxidant elimination of free radicals, the dangerous by-product of oxygen metabolism. The FDA and various long-term scientific and medical studies have been conducted on the effects of selenium upon cancer, AIDS, and heart disease;

a preponderance of these studies have shown encouraging results. The FDA recommends that an adult daily intake not exceed 400 micrograms (mcg) as excessive selenium intake can be toxic. Various foods have good amounts of selenium, such as Brazil nuts (though this source can have strong amounts that may exceed the FDA daily allowance recommendation), tuna, beef, cod, turkey, chicken breast, pastas, oatmeal, cottage cheese, eggs, rice, etc.

Selenium supplements of an organic source (not containing inorganic sodium selenite and sodium selenate of a dosage of 200 mcg a day can be a very strong immune and antioxidant booster. Selenium has also been shown to reduce the effects of chemotherapy, a strong antidisease preventive measure, and antitumor fighter.

I will try selenium supplements. I may continuing my research on multivitamin supplements and will have more to report on this perhaps in my next weekly diary entry.

I spent much of the day reading both online materials and books and articles. The refrigerator repair per MW man came by at 2:00 PM and found that my thermostat had gone off, probably after the freezer door had not properly shut this past weekend, and so the entire refrigerator had shut down and only reset itself after I closed the freezer door shut midweek. So no repair was needed, but he did do a diagnostic checkup. Whew, glad that is solved.

My amp-receiver had to be returned to the repair shop. I upgraded by turntable to a modern one and gave my Technics turntable of thirty years to Joseph Yoon who has been developing his DJ skills. But my amp-receiver of twenty years has some glitches, and I hope it can be fixed. I'm a low-tech person (yes, I'm a Luddite and proud to be one!) and don't throw away machines if they can be repaired and repaired again, until they are finally totally obsolete (parts unable to be found anymore) or thoroughly dead. I love my many LPs, so I'm anxious to have my system back to working order soon.

My day finally came to a relaxing end by 5:00 PM. I found my corner CD-video-DVD street vendor had the latest copy of the DVD *Mission: Impossible 3* and got it for $5 and had an entertaining early evening before going to sleep around 11:30 PM.

November 18, 2006

This is the first Saturday of my chemo cycle that I'm not totally wiped out and filled with nausea. I also didn't feel the need to take any Benadryl any of the past two nights.

I got up at 6:30 AM feeling rested and not able to sleep anymore. I should be mindful and not push myself and have an easy day. Glad the refrigerator-freezer is working again, so I can get some groceries.

I juiced some apples, pears, and kiwis this morning. There is nothing better than squeezing your own juice. I recommend the Breville juicer. It is simply the *best* home juicer on the market because (1) it has a huge mouth, and you don't have to peel anything and can put entire apples into it with slicing; (2) it's got a 3/4 to 1 horsepower motor, very powerful; (3) it's got a huge waste container to collect all rinds, seeds, skins, peels, etc; (4) it's got a large juice canister and strainer so what you get is total juice and separated pulp.

I use the pulp to make sauces and marinades, and for those of you with gardens, you can use the waste for great composting!

Because I have been drinking a lot of juices, my glucose level has risen above normal. I'm not too concerned with this. All my blood tests have been very good, with normal white and red cell counts (though the white has been dropping, but not yet into a dangerous zone that would seriously compromise my immune system and therefore require I stop eating raw produce and fish for its possible increased bacteria) and platelets. My blood is tested weekly to watch for any dangerous falls or elevations in my chemistry.

So far today, Saturday, the last day of chemo cycle number 4, the worst side effect has been increased peripheral neuropathy. My feet and hands react to any coldness, from bare feet touching granite floors, to my hands going into a refrigerator, to breathing in cold air. My extremities get numb, and I lose coordination and dexterity. I have to wear clothes and thick socks inside my home and sometimes when I go to bed. But the nausea and fatigue aren't as bad these past three days.

DIARY 6: REAL DRAGONS FLY!

November 19–28, 2006

This was a nonchemo week. While I had little nausea after my last chemo session on November 16, 2006, I was smashed by the worse diarrhea I've had so far since beginning chemo. For almost five days, from late Tuesday night, November 21, 2006, to Saturday evening, November 25, 2006, I was very sick. I was able to take a few hours on Thursday, November 23, 2006, to spend Thanksgiving over at Ann T. Greene and Mark O'Ferrall's place. Since my stomach was completely empty, I was able to eat and enjoy the meal, but as soon as I got home, it all left my stomach.

A possible reason for this really bad diarrhea is that my refrigerator-freezer is still broken and not keeping things cold or frozen. Probably I ate some spoiled food during the week. I again had to throw out a lot of food. Because it is the holidays, I can't get a repair person to come in until next week. So I'll just buy food daily and not save anything. Perhaps this is preparation for a nontechnological lifestyle should I decide to exit modern civilization and not have any refrigeration devices anymore.

So far all my blood counts have been very good. While they have fallen, which is what the chemo will do by killing off all new cells, they have not fallen into any danger zones. My blood counts need to be closely and regularly monitored. Should they fall into the danger zone, I will need medication to boost them up.

At my last chemo session at the hospital, my surgically installed Medi-port (the conduit put into my chest to allow blood to be drawn or for chemo drugs to be infused) was clogged, and it took over an hour to unclog it. I have to now take daily a 1 mg dosage of Coumadin to prevent the Medi-port from clogging. Clogging typically happens to devices that are installed in a human body. Coumadin is a dangerous drug, though the dosage I'm taking is very small, but my liver function has to be carefully watched as well as the interaction with other drugs. Coumadin is used a lot to prevent artery clogging.

The day after Thanksgiving, my sister Florence and her family visited me. My nephew, Ethan, who is fourteen, has been studying the Korean martial art tae kwon do, and is getting very good. He can do one-arm push-ups, just like his Uncle Fred!

My sister Florence and her husband, Mark, both of whom are physicians, noted that colon cancer over the past one hundred years has dropped in per capita incidence, possibly due to refrigeration. People in the early part of the twentieth century ate food that was often spoiled and not good because refrigeration wasn't available or too expensive.

Florence and Mark recommended that I research "oral rehydration fluids" that I can make myself to prevent dehydration and to restore my electrolytes lost from the diarrhea. One out of six people in the world suffer from lack of clean drinking water. Because they are in the third world, buying Gatorade is too expensive. A simple formula is using 1 liter of *clean* water or boiled water (then cooled) combined with one teaspoon of common household salt, one-fourth teaspoon of baking soda, and four to eight teaspoons of white sugar (or better, molasses). The main thing you need to replenish is salt, sugar (glucose), and potassium. Eating a BRAT diet (banana-rice-apple sauce-tea) helps. But the best thing I found suggested to me by my sister Flora (who struggled with cervical cancer and had bad side effects from both chemo and radiation therapies) is to drink the gruel from a small amount of boiled rice with five cups of water. This is like Chinese congee (rice porridge gruel). During the worst diarrhea, this was the only thing that could stay in my stomach.

Congee is very common in China, particularly in poor rural areas. It is simply rice with extra water boiled and ginger, garlic, scallions, other vegetables, seafood, meats all can be added for a very nutritious meal that loosens phlegm and congestion (great on cold days or when you have the flu or cold: it is the Chinese equivalent of chicken soup). Many Chinatown eateries serve congee.

I read with great interest Dr. Ralph Moss's website e-mailed to me by visual artist-professor Beverly Naidus (www.cancerdecisions. com). I agree that the CAM (complementary and alternative medicine) movement has gotten short shrift here in the United States. I also think there are a lot of scams and false promises within the CAM movement as well. Moss, while pro-CAM and critical of a lot of the mainstream medical establishment, still shares and upholds with the mainstream establishment that a cure for cancer can be found. I am of the belief that a cure will be impossible because it is part of the very fabric of industrial society. There is no single cause; there can be no single cure. Billions and billions of dollars have been raised and allocated to the cure industry, with no progress in any substantial way. While I'm inclined to believe that cancer predates industrialization, I believe it is magnified and exacerbated by industrialism's rampant environmental toxicity, including the pervasiveness of electromagnetic radiation generated from all electronic technology from electric lights to cell phone radiation.

I believe a societal detoxification would include repairing the ozone layer, significant reduction in all electromagnetic radiation, a massive change in food production, and elimination of fossil fuels. Without these measures, cancer won't be effectively fought. The expectation that a miracle drug will be invented, or a single potent treatment, is illogical as well as fundamentally unscientific.

Part of the battle on the food production front involves the choices we make about our diet. Something that Beverly Naidus shared with me is the health-beneficial role of fermented food, especially tofu (fermented soybean):

> Tofu is one of the excellent fermented foods, as is *umeboshi* plum, miso, *natto*, shoyu, *tamari*, *kombucha*, etc. It's no wonder that the Japanese have the lowest cancer stats. Kefir, vinegar, sauerkraut, yogurt, wine, and brewers yeast are all useful to add to that probiotic diet as well.

One Chinese herbal treatment, *juzentaihoto* (or JT-48 or JTT), has been recognized even by sectors of the Western medical establishment as having efficacy in treating the harsh side effects of chemotherapy as well as in AIDs and other serious ailments. However, I can't seem to find out where to get these herbs. If anyone reading this has a special connection to an herbalist or Chinese medicine specialist and can help me locate how to get this herb, please get in touch.

On Sunday, November 26, 2006, the diarrhea was gone, and I felt a lot better. Since then, I have daily been practicing the sax and find I'm playing better than ever. I also continue to exercise, spending a lot of time on lower back and abdominal exercises since the days I'm sick, I'm on my back a lot. I try to walk at least one mile a day.

Jocelyn Clark from Juneau, Alaska, and leader of IIIZ+ (Three Z Plus), a unique chamber ensemble of three Asian zithers (Korean *kumungo*, Japanese *koto* and Chinese *guzheng* plus percussionist), a group that commissioned me to compose "Suite for Matriarchal Shaman Warriors," sent me disks of their performance of my piece from their fall tour of Boston, Massachusetts, and Germany. I was thrilled to hear how well they performed the piece and hope someday they can record it. www.iiiz.jocelynclark.com.

I only have Sunday through Wednesday as good days before my next chemo treatment on Thursday, November 30, 2006. I'm hoping I can use this time to begin composing my American Composers Orchestra commission, which I've titled "When the Real Dragons Fly" taken from the famous Ho Chi Minh quote, "When the prison doors open, the real dragons will fly."

November 30 to December 13, 2006
Week 5 of Chemo

This time, my Benadryl dosage for the final infusion of 5FU (fluorouracil) was lowered to 25 mg instead of the 100 mg given last time, which really knocked me, turning me into a groggy sleepwalker. I napped for about forty-five minutes, woke up to pee, and noticed the time was 3:00 PM and was ready to be driven home by Cristian Amigo, who spent the day with me at the treatment center. I came home fully awake. Since my refrigerator-freezer is not working, Cristian and I had dinner at Antek, a great local Polish diner (cheap prices and good, stick-to-your bones food). I didn't suffer from the extreme drowsiness and didn't have to go right to bed.

This chemo session has been the mildest with only fatigue and one day of diarrhea (thankfully).

During the dark days of diarrhea during chemo session number 4, I couldn't do much except lie on the coach and watch DVDs. I have been seeing the future as depicted in U.S. popular culture via TV (viewable in the *Star Trek* original series DVD collection, the *Star Trek: Enterprise* four-season DVD collection, and the new *Battlestar Galactica* DVD series), and contrary to fans and most interpretations, it is a future that I interpret to be bleak and what I would not endorse.

Most would interpret *Star Trek* creator Gene Roddenberry's vision of humanity's future to be very optimistic. After breaking the barrier of light speed, supposedly humanity will become united, eliminate war, poverty, inequality, racism and sexism, most diseases, greed, and even do away with money! People will do things for self-improvement and the betterment of society. Sounds like utopian communism!

But this Star Trekian future contains vast, powerful empires (Klingon, Romulan, Cardassian, Breen, Dominion, Borg—and possibly others that exist in areas of our galaxy for which the Terran-centric Star Fleet and United Federation of Planets haven't gotten to yet), all involved in dangerous skirmishes, even outright galactic war, with incredible weapons of mass destruction that make our atomic weapons seem like bows and arrows and spears. Furthermore, Star Fleet and the United Federation of Planets, Earth-led and created entities, rely upon a vast and powerful military component, have extremely stratified ranking and hierarchy (admirals and commodores at the top, then captains and officers, civilians seem to be nobodies unless they are ambassadors, and officials given authority by the United Federation of Planets, which is something of a galactic UN, analogously and equally ineffective and subordinate to Star Fleet/the United States, though the propaganda is that Star Fleet/the United States is subordinate to the United Federation of Planets/UN (but when does the United States ever abide by the UN in reality?).

Domestically, on Earth, natural disasters such as the possibility of a Hurricane Katrina, seem to be solved by technology in the Roddenberry Earth of the twenty-third century. In the movie, *Star Trek 4* (the one with bringing back humpback whales from the twentieth century to the twenty-third century, after they were killed to extinction but are needed to communicate to a powerful interstellar probe that is depleting Earth's oceans and blocking the sun), we learn that most disastrous weather phenomenon is curtailed and controlled by a planetwide weather net. Social problems, rarely discussed in any amount of detail or depth, have been assumed to have withered away by a heightened global consciousness inspired by the possibilities of interstellar contact and the technological breakthrough of faster-than-light speed travel. (Though vestiges of racist thinking and attitudes continue with xenophobia and terran species centrism expressed in the original series opener "Where no *man* has gone before," which was changed by *The Next Generation* series to "Where no one has gone before" or expressions such as "inalienable human rights," etc. Cultural interspecies conflicts and misunderstandings have been common tropes in many *Star Trek* episodes.)

Despite all this progress, however, Star Fleet and the UFP are huge bureaucracies that, admittedly, can't avoid problems of personal ambition, political favoritism and opportunism and careerism, jealousy, competition, rivalry, egomania, indifference, and benign neglect: that human personal flaws are magnified by the power of hierarchal organization and can be insidious and malevolent. A structural critique of capitalism, industrialism, technocracy, and class society in general is avoided, though it seems that genetic engineering (fictionalized in a Eugenics War and the dangerous hubris of constructing genetically superior humanoids) is opposed, primarily from a moral premise of tampering with nature and playing at God. No stories or discussions focus on the more daily manifestations of genetic engineering through genetically modified organisms found common in processed foods, stem cell research, etc. Nor is the deeper issue of Promethean progress ever challenged: is building something faster, bigger, stronger, more powerful really *better*? Or will this progress obsolesce other organic traits, traditions, and talents?

It seems that the media entertainment depiction of our future's continuing problems are the result of human nature (hubris, ambition, flawed decision-making, jealousy, etc), which are controlled by extensive codes, regulations, and hierarchal authoritative bodies (including the United Federation of Planets' Prime Directive in the natural development of a planet or society). Science fiction, like all arts that seek marketplace legitimacy and acceptance, can't be too controversial or radical if they are to be approved by corporate gatekeepers who may deem some subject matter too heretical to return a profit.

A completely militarized future is the premise of *Battlestar Galactica*. But instead of wars with extraterrestrials, it is Armageddon between humans (the only species so far evident in the cosmos) and the Cyclones (the machines created by humans who rebelled and now seek the extermination of their once masters-creators). The interesting conundrum: who's worse, the humans or the machines? In an interesting twist, the machines have accepted a monotheistic faith (resembling Christianity) in their crusade to subjugate humanity to it. And humanity is polytheistic (an amalgam of Greco-Roman gods and mythology). Given that humanity has been reduced to a population of less than fifty thousand, in perpetual exile, loosely bound together in a fleet of large space-traveling ships, issues of production and socioeconomic matters are largely avoided or are part of the willing suspension-of-disbelief one needs to accept in order to accept the dramatic plausibility of the overall premise of this reality. Major tropes in the *Battlestar Galactica* series are individual moral and character challenges raised by military conflict: loyalty to duty versus individual moral conscience, does the means justify the ends, pragmatism versus idealism, etc.

In both the *Star Trek* and the *Battlestar Galactica* franchises, the Other exists as the antagonist (whether these Others be aliens or Cyclones). In the short-lived *Firefly* series, the known cosmos has no aliens, no

"Other" except marginalized humans. In *Firefly*, five hundred years in the future, the last remaining superpowers on Earth were China and the United States and a hybridized culture has developed (in which American characters speak Chinese slang), and humans have ventured into space to colonized habitable worlds as part of the new frontier, but never encountering any other intelligent life-forms. Human social relations have extended into a socioeconomic interplanetary apartheid of core planets, which are affluent megalopolises, and the border planets, which are the hinterland Bantustans. A recent rebellion by the border planets was defeated, thereby hardening inequality.

In *Star Trek*, the basic premise is that technology can take us to the stars, but our human nature is oftentimes less advanced and remains the source of our flaws and hindrances. Also embedded in the *Star Trek* outlook is that technology is the engine that solved our social problems (without giving any details on how this happened except a cursory assumption about a "great awakening" of human consciousness). The major problem I have is that without social revolution, technology primarily benefits the controlling and exploiting classes. Capitalism, and its consequent industrialization of the planet, is a powerful productive engine, transcending the previous problems of scarcity and human subordination to biology nature, into a global force that has the possibility of eliminating scarcity (feeding, clothing, and providing for all humans) and dominating nature (even destroying the planet both from human-designed energies and from pollution/toxicity and environmental damage from the by-products of human industrialization). Capitalism's primary contradiction is that it creates more problems than it can solve. As long as a social system exists in which the pursuit of profit and individualism preempts social equity and justice and the health of the planet, then technology will only serve to exacerbate and intensify inequality, injustice, and ecocide.

In *Battlestar Galactica*, exploited labor is not eliminated, only transferred to intelligent robots who later become sentient and self-aware enough to rebel and even engineer their own cybernetic evolutionary offspring who look, feel, taste, love, and emote like humans. And from all indications, this next-generation of human–machine life-form seems as iniquitous as their human originals. Resources are overwhelmingly expended in the conflict over who will be master and who will be slave.

In *Firefly*, an interplanetary fascist police state and its attendant black market economies, gangsters, underground subcultures, etc., while perhaps more socially variegated and textured than the realities of *Star Trek* or *Battlestar Galactica*, nonetheless maintain that class division and stratification is immutable, inevitable, and natural.

So commercial media science fiction, while dramatically compelling, nonetheless reinforce and underscore the dominant worldview of bourgeois class society that human nature (our good and bad aspects) will persist unchanged, including aggression, greed, egotism, hubris, and will continue to drive humans to dominate, control, and rule over Others, ourselves, and nature.

Thank you for allowing me to share with you my philosophical contemplations. Please use the Warriors for Fred LISTSERV to add your own opinions. In future journal entries, I will attempt to connect my growing beliefs in Ludditism with matters of personal, societal, and planetary health.

THE ONGOING STRUGGLE TO FIX MY REFRIGERATOR

I have been without a working refrigerator for almost six weeks due to the bureaucratic ineffectualness of Frigidaire and its service subcontractors. I have had three repair companies referred by Frigidaire, giving me four different diagnoses as to what is wrong and what needs to be done. Two of three were incompetent and unconcerned about service quality and took the majority of the five weeks of delays and unresponsiveness. I have registered complaints against them: Harp Home Services and Herb's Appliance. The third one, Dial Appliance Service, while prompt, sent two different repair people who had two different diagnoses. The last repair person stated that my refrigerator had an internal Freon leak and was unrepairable.

I contacted F-EMA and reported this last diagnosis (which I suspect to be correct). F-EMA verified this from Dial Appliance Service. They have now referred my case to their replacement authorization division to rule on whether I should be given a completely new, comparable refrigerator. The wait continues.

I *urge* everyone *not* to buy Frigidaire home appliances but consider a company like Sears, which has its own internal repair services instead of subcontracting to parasitic subcontractors who profit from delays, repeated visits that don't accomplish anything (which they bill for), all of which they try to milk the corporate teat. This is like the disconnected multipayer health care system we have in the United States in which a multitude of insurance companies profiteer off the fragmentation and disconnection of specialists, hospitals, multiple billing, unnecessary and repeated tests, lack of centralized records, billing and medical files, making waste, inefficiency, bureaucracy, parasitism, and incompetence rampant, while integrity, excellence, responsiveness, and genuine concern are in short shrift.

By next week I will know whether Frigidaire will replace my refrigerator or I will simply dump the one I have and go to Sears and get a new one.

Thank you to all my friends who have come by and driven me to Flushing Chinatown and elsewhere for delicious meals during this ordeal.

DIARY 7: THE IRRESISTABLE DIALECTIC

December 14–28, 2006

I've reached my midway point, six out of twelve chemo sessions, or three out of six months of treatment. This session was the smoothest: no allergic reaction for the 5FU infusion, except a tinge of nausea and the 25 mgs of Benadryl made me sleep for forty-five minutes.

Thanks to Taylor Ho Bynum for driving me to this chemo session, staying with me and driving me home afterward (but before we went home, we stopped in Flushing Chinatown at a great Hunan-Szechuan restaurant called "Tasty and Spicy," which I learned about by reading a rave *New York Times'* restaurant review on November 30, 2006).

And thanks to one of my longest and dearest friends, Gwen Mok, a piano professor at San Jose State University, who flew out from California to be with me for this chemo session and to be my trouble shooting enforcer by calling Frigidaire-Electrolux and getting them to finally promise to getting me a brand-new replacement refrigerator. Hopefully, before Christmas, I'll have a working refrigerator, and I can rejoin civilized modern society!

My main side effects so far with this session of chemo has been some intermittent hiccups, passing gas, fatigue, mild redness on my chest and back (hives) from my allergic reaction to the 5FU drug, and very short periods of peripheral neuropathy (numbness of my extremities triggered by cold). While the harshness of the chemo seems to have diminished, I find myself with greater lengths of fatigue and less full energy days as I had during earlier chemo sessions. My sister Flora, who fought cervical cancer twice, tells me that as chemo goes on, I will get more tired and require more rest.

Some difficult and painful news. My friend Molly Sturges, a fabulous singer-songwriter, co-leader of the band Bing!, with her husband, saxophonist Chris Jonas (former founding member of the Brooklyn Sax Quartet), was diagnosed with tongue cancer two weeks ago and underwent surgery on Monday, December 11, 2006. Fortunately, she is in stage 1. My love and support goes out to her. We have talked on the phone and will continue to talk as I share my war experiences.

All my blood counts continue to be good. My glucose, which for the last two week was very high at 213–214 (normal is between 80–99) and which generated concern that I might have a tendency toward diabetes, this time tested at 117. Dr. Patel and others believe that the steroid, Decadron, that I take for three days postchemo, elevates my glucose, and it should be fine when I complete the chemo treatments.

My weight is now hovering around 218, and my blood pressure has increased. On December 14, 2006, I had four blood pressure readings: the first was 174/130 (astronomically too high!); then 150/110; then 148/104; and finally, 130/80 (much better). Several factors could account for these high numbers: my weight gain, lack of exercise this past week due to bad weather outside and time consumed in fighting for my refrigerator repair, and the overall stress from this ordeal. I intend to exercise more from now on, but the constant fatigue has left me with considerably less energy than I had before during the earlier chemo phase.

Part of what has helped me interrupt the stress of my refrigerator struggle has been completing my composition commission "When the Real Dragons Fly!" for the American Composers Orchestra. I finished on December 11, 2006 and have started hand copying the instrumental parts. The work is based on a traditional Chinese folksong called "Soong Lang," which was used as a farewell song. I rework the concept of "farewell" to mean farewell to political imprisonment, farewell to the prison industrial complex, and farewell to U.S. imperialism! It is a concerto for baritone saxophone for medium-size orchestra. It premieres February 8, 2008, at Zankel Hall in Carnegie Hall and then travels to Philadelphia (University of Philadelphia Annenberg Center). The commission was championed by the great composer-antiwar/ peace activist Derek Bermel whose own CD *Soul Garden* on CRI is one of my all-time favorite recordings! Please check it out, incredible orchestrations and very soulful writing and brilliant performances by the instrumentalists.

Some more good news: Chamber Music America has given Purdue University's American Studies Department headed by comrade-scholar Dr. Bill Mullen $7,500 to present in concert my Afro Asian Music Ensemble. With Joseph Yoon, the band's agent-manager, we will build a U.S. tour for early 2008. We will combine the tour with the launch and celebration of the publication of the new anthology *Afro Asia: Revolutionary Political and Cultural Connections between* African Americans and Asian Americans (Duke University Press), co-edited by myself and Bill Mullen. The tour will coincide with my first year anniversary of finishing chemotherapy treatment (hopefully one year of being cancer free!).

Some more good news: Elaine Fong, artistic and executive director of Odaiko New England, one of America's daring Asian American *taiko* drum-percussion ensemble, will commission me to compose a new work called "The Wild, Wild East Suite" for 2008–2009. I am very excited about creating a new and challenging work that will extend beyond heretofore practices of *taiko* drumming (for example, from unison rhythms and duple meter to multiple polyrhythms and triple meter, greater complexity of texture).

I have resolved in my work as a composer to write music for the most unusual and unique ensembles. So many other composers write for the conventional string quartets, wind and brass ensembles and orchestra works, and they are great at that. I believe my calling is to compose for the unconventional. Should a mainstream ensemble be courageous and committed enough to commission me to write for them, I won't turn them down provided they allow me complete freedom and discretion in the political/narrative and aesthetic concept. As everyone knows, I am *very* easy to work with as long as integrity is the primary operative principle.

Peggy Choy has also applied to the University of Wisconsin-Madison to have me as artist-in-residence for spring 2008 to teach multicultural performance/collaboration, to compose new works for her, to have my Afro Asian Music Ensemble perform and do residency activities, and to speak on panels to students and faculty.

I spent the Christmas holiday with my family at my sister Florence's home in Maryland outside of Washington, D.C. My youngest sister Flora and her daughter, Emma (eight years old), flew from the Bay Area to NYC. Flora picked me up and drove us to DC in a rental car where I spent four wonderful days with my sisters, their children, my brother-in-laws, and my mother. My sisters Florence and Flora drove me back to NYC on December 26, 2006 to get ready for my upcoming chemo session number 7 for December 28, 2006.

WHY I'M A MARXIST MATRIARCHAL LUDDITE

I'm a Marxist because I believe class analysis is how to fundamentally understand the interconnection of power, exploitation, oppression; that while it is helpful to change individuals, policies and practices, that without fundamental systemic change, it will only be cosmetic reform and not revolutionary transformation.

I'm a matriarchalist because I believe that the class system we have had for the past five thousand to eight years of human history has been systems of minority patriarchal rule of the owners of land, property, and labor *over* the majority. A new era in humanity will mean the end of that dominance and the return of rule to the majority of producers. Since women bear 100 percent of the world's children, do 70 percent of the world's work (albeit un- or underpaid), grow 60 percent of the world's food, but earn 10 percent of the world's income and own less than 1 percent of the world's property, the *reversal* of this order will be matriarchy.

I'm a Luddite because I'm *not* antitechnology, but for *low* technology. Low impact upon the environment and restricting and eliminating technology used for social repression, exploitation, dispossession of workers' control and human degradation, dependency, and fragmentation. The solution to halting and reversing ecological destruction and social inequality and injustice will mean a fundamental alteration of our current relations and trend of consumption in which the United States, 5 to 6 percent of the world's population, continues to consume 50 percent of the world's resources with hugely disproportionate waste, pollution, and depletion of nonrenewable resources.

We as individuals can alter our lifestyle consumption, live with less (not more), change what and how we consume, but we must also seize control of society so that the biggest culprits of waste, exploitation, and consumption (mostly the corporate behemoths) won't continue their wanton ways. That is the irresistible dialectic: the reciprocity of changing both individuals' consciousness and practices and the system.

Thank you for allowing me to share my philosophical contemplations. Feel free to contribute your own.

DIARY 8: FIGHTING THE BATTLE OF JERICHO

December 28, 2006 to January 11, 2007

The extreme ups and downs of the early chemo sessions have flattened out. My first eight weeks of chemo had very bad days of nausea, diarrhea, and great fatigue, as well as very good days where I felt full of energy and could exercise at almost previous precancer peak levels. Now, while not showing the worst side effects of nausea and diarrhea, I have a lot less energy and days seem to be filled with a mild fatigue that inhibits the bursts of energy I previously had.

My sister Flora, who fought two wars against cervical cancer (first appearing in 2000 and then reoccurring in 2004), tells me that as she progressed in her chemo and radiation treatments, all she could do was rest and sleep as the fatigue was considerable.

On December 18, 2006, I finally got a new refrigerator (a Westinghouse) replacing my broken Frigidaire-Electrolux. After a six-week ordeal of incompetent and unresponsive service companies referred by Frigidaire-Electrolux, it was finally determined that the broken refrigerator was unrepairable due to an internal Freon gas leak. Freon was banned in all new refrigerators manufactured and sold in the United States by the federal government as part of stemming greenhouse gas emission during the late 1990s. While existing Freon refrigerators continued to be sold, the new ones, I'm told by the manager at P. C. Richards where I bought my refrigerator, are a lot lower quality and even a $4,000 to $5,000 subzero will last anywhere from three to seven years now. The extended ten-year warranty for $300 is a must to cover repair labor, parts, and even the replacement of a new comparable refrigerator should it not be repairable. At last the ordeal is over. I called Access-A-Ride to make a trip over to Trader Joe's the next day!

My doctors tell me that my body is adjusting (getting used to) the accumulation of chemo drugs and that is why I'm experiencing less hills and valleys and a more overall, general fatigue. I'm now needing to sleep and rest a lot more. Some days I'm awake and active for only six hours.

My blood cell counts are all doing very well, even occasionally increasing in numbers! I attribute this to the careful and concerted nutritional effort: a variety of raw fruits and vegetables, very low sodium, low fat, the elimination of all beef- and cow-related food (e.g., cow's milk and extremely minimal use of butter only in cooking, not spreading on top of food), complex carbs, the elimination of white refined sugar and white bleached flour, a variety of fruit juices, teas, water. Cancer fighting and at the cellular level is a combination of the medical front waged by chemo and your doctors and the personal front waged by the tri-combination of oxygenation-hydration-nutrition, which seems to be working well for me.

A VERY SPECIAL SURPRISE EVENT, JANUARY 6, 2007, AT THE BAMCafé

My friend, the curator Limor Tomer, had recently left her position of many years at the BAMCafé. She contacted me via e-mail to invite me to her going-away party as she recently took on the position as head of programming at WNYC radio. Limor e-mailed me and said it would mean a lot to her if I came to her going away party at the BAMCafé, and I said I would. That Saturday, I slept for most of the day, overslept, rushed to get dressed and hail a cab to get over to BAM. As I was walking in, I noticed a lot of people I knew but just thought that they were also there to celebrate Limor. I was escorted to a seat with Joe Melillo, Pat Scully, and Alice Bernstein and didn't think much of it. Joe Melillo handed me a program that read "A Celebration Tribute for Fred Ho," and I thought he was pulling my leg, a practical joke. I only realized what the event truly was when Magdalena Gómez got up and emceed the event explicitly stating it was for me.

I was surprised and shocked! I hadn't expected this at all. And what a terrific evening. So many great artists performed that spanned forms and cultural expressions from Eastern Europe, Iran, Egypt, Hawaii, the Americas (both hemispheres), Africa/African America, Asia/Asian America, the traditional to the avant-garde. Everyone was blown away, both audience and artists, with the whole program. Thank you so much to the performers!

And thank you to Limor, everyone at BAM who made the event possible. Joe Melillo spoke at the end and handed me a check to match the monies that all the performers had kicked back to me by declining their artist fees. I was very moved by the outpouring of love and support. As a friend remarked, it is rare that an institution can be so human and do something as loving and generous in friendship.

BAM has been my performance home in New York since 1997, a decade ago. The place has a very special place in my development and identity: not only for its special-ness to my home of Brooklyn, but for its role in adventurous, daring, bold and risk-taking creative work, set by Next Wave festival founder Harvey Lichtenstein. BAM and I are an organic, natural "match" and walking into the place whether it is to rehearse, attend an event, see a movie, eat and catch a performance at the BAMCafé, meet with the staff—it feels like I'm walking into "my" place. From the security guards, to the stage hands, to the staff, we all know each other, stop to say hi and chat.

Thank you to everyone who was part of this evening, especially to Magdalena Gómez who stealthily organized the whole program. I shall remember this special event for the rest of my life, which will be a long one!

The First Two Weeks in January 2007

I continue to have many visitors, both local and out of town, coming over to visit me.

Quincy and Margaret Troupe visited the day after New Year's bringing some fabulous black beans, rice, and ratatouille. We discussed resuming work on our opera, *Mr. Mystery: The Return of Sun Ra to Save Planet Earth!* Limor Tomer, curator of performances at the Whitney Museum, called to book a stage reading of excerpts from the book-libretto this summer at the museum at Seventh-fifth Street and Madison Avenue.

Thank-yous to Jayne Cortez for sending me her latest CD anthology of her selected hits from over the past two decades; to literary agent Frances Goldin's financial gift of $100; to saxophonist-composer Ned Rothenberg for giving me his new CD *Internal Diaspora*, which is a musical gem.

One of my longest musical friends and mutual minds Hafez Modirzadeh, who is Iranian American, dropped by for an afternoon to discuss his latest philosophical epiphany described as "DisIntegrationism": to paraphrase, the need for counterhegemonic discourses, ideas and creative expressionisms to not only be totally oppositional, but also to aggressively dismantle and extricate, in order to begin to construct as much as possible from a *tabula rasa* basis.

While Hafez has never been one to discount the importance of traditions (being both an ethnomusicologist by training and investigative scholarship, and as someone who plays the tenor saxophone evoking the great masters), he, nonetheless, to his unique credit, recognizes how much tradition can also contain baggage and conservatism. In his in-depth study and appreciation of the late great martial artist Bruce Lee's syncretic philosophy of *Jeet Kune Do* (the way of the intercepting fist), we share the concept that the goal of developing and mastering technique is to have *no* technique. That formic activity must become intuition.

For me the point of musical mastery is to develop our chi (life force energy) to change the world): in the ethos and exertion expressed in the African American spiritual (slave) song: "Joshua fought the battle of Jericho, and [by playing his trumpet] the walls come tumbling down." I'm looking for musicians who want to bring down the walls of Jericho with their sound.

Not since the great George Russell's Lydian Chromatic concept developed in the 1950s has anyone made a theoretical breakthrough in jazz improvisation as Hafez's chromodal discourse theory, which he developed in the 1980s. This theory is a profound, polysemous conception of cross-cultural improvisation that propounds the necessity of reciprocal cultural transgressions if true interactivity and mutual discourse is to happen. For example, technically Hafez, through alternative fingerings for the tenor saxophone, is able to play a Persian temperament (tunings) to the dominant western European diatonic (half-and-whole steps, the black and white keys on a piano) scale by producing quarter tones (pitches in between the half steps, so think of a piano now having "blue" keys in between not only the black and white keys). While African American music, and most hybrid music that combine variable pitched and fixed pitch relations (described in

African American music as the "blue notes") as a result of cross-cultural interactions over social and temporal space (African-and-white/ European American settler colonial historical dynamic of segregation and miscegenation), Hafez has systematized this musical hybridity in regard to pitch in his chromodal discourse theory. Quite revolutionary.

Joseph Franklin and Laurel Wycoff, from Albuquerque, New Mexico, also stopped by for an afternoon of Japanese lunch and long conversations. Joseph has published a memoir of his life in American new music, titled *Settling Scores*. It is an illuminating and enjoyable read about important years when mavericks, upstarts, iconoclasts, avant-gardists, experimentalists, and musicians and composers who didn't want to follow the staid legacy and practices of western European concert music practices, traditions, and institutions banded together and became a movement in American culture from the late 1950s (rebellion against Eisenhower-ism and the mass culturing of America, socially/philosophically/psychosexually critique by Herbert Marcuse, among many others) through the 1980s and early 1990s. It looks at their/our successes and failures, our dreams and mistakes, as well as our enemies and opposition who sought to undermine, derail and eventually succeeded to some degree of marginalizing "new music." I am reminded constantly by something Mao proffered: external contradictions become operative through internal ones, which Mao simply understood from Sun Tsu—"Know thy enemy, know thy self, 100 battles, 100 victories."

Peggy Choy, Korean American choreographer-dancer, cultural theorist, and Asian American movement activist, who grew up in Hawaii and now teaches at the University of Wisconsin–Madison, came into town to hold auditions and begin rehearsals on her new work, *Gateless Gate: Women of the Scarred Earth*. I love the concept/title of "gateless gate," a revolutionary Zen notion: we need standards of excellence, selectivity, a vanguard, but it must not be exclusionary, in-group, incestuous, self-perpetuating, and self-preserving—something like a "leaderless leadership." Or as Isadora Duncan, the revolutionary and iconoclastic choreographer almost a century ago said, "I don't want to join a party that can't party and dance." It is that profound, revolutionary combination/unity of humility, and confidence, power and humbleness, decisiveness and openness to listen and incorporate, of collectivity and command. This is the area of self-transformation, of the role of individuality in collective movements and communities, the so-called spiritual. People empowered to be their own leaders and yet scientific, imaginative, and disciplined enough to function cooperatively and collectively on a larger societal and global level. Peggy made a big pot of miso soup for me and joined me, along with my step-aunt and step-uncle Wolhee Choe and Bob Hawks, to my chemo session number 8.

Thank you to Paget Walker for driving me to my doctor's visit and spending several hours hanging out and talking with me. If I forgot to mention anyone else's visits, I apologize. Just use the listserv and write in with your story and commentary.

Please come to the staged reading of *Dragon vs. Eagle* at the Apollo Theater Salon (black box second floor), 253 West 125th Street, Harlem. Seven terrific actors will read from the script/book to preview and try out my latest collaboration with Ruth Margraff, the third in the *Voice of the Dragon* trilogy. The event is *free*. If you want to risk showing up at the door, please come a bit early as seating is limited.

Here is just a short description of the story:

In a time and place beyond history and fantasy, an Eagle Empire has arisen to occupy the globe with its monopolist and megacorporate conquistadors. New lethal gladiators of supersteroidal and genetically enhanced omnipotence crush all competition with the zealotry of a crusade. Under the Eagle's eclipsing wingspan, one man, in the land of the Dragons, turns to the cult of atavism. One disaster of the mythic Shaolin Temple gets remastered from its darkest hour. One villain, once invincible, gets resurrected as the quintessential warrior in the battle of the centuries against an unstoppable onslaught—the titanic clash of dragon versus eagle.

DIARY 9: THE RESULTS OF YOUR LOVE AND SUPPORT

Chemo Session Number 8 (Four More to Go Until March 10, 2007!)
January 11, 2007

My good friend Peggy Choy joined my step-aunt and step-uncle Wolhee Choe and Bob Hawks to this chemo session. My treatment team is figuring out how to best ease my allergic reaction to the third of the three chemo drugs, the 5FU (fluorouracil), and this session was the mildest.

I am definitely feeling the accumulation of the chemo drugs as I am very fatigued and am sleeping a lot more than in the early stages of my treatment. There are some days when I'm only awake for seven hours a day. It seems heavier fatigue is the main side effect. Almost gone are nausea and diarrhea. However, the peripheral neuropathy has worsened. Even in my well-heated apartment, I have to wear two layers of socks and slippers on my feet and gloves on my hands.

Thank you to all of you who continue to send me cards, e-mails, care packages, and donations. And to those of you who come by with cars to take me to and from my doctor's appointments, or bring me out to lunch or dinner. A growing group of us have been discovering the culinary wonders of Flushing Chinatown. The Chinatowns of Lower Manhattan and Sunset Park, Brooklyn, are much more Cantonese-Fukienese based (southern Chinese) while Flushing is more diverse, both in terms of Chinese regions (e.g., Taiwan, Shanghai, Hunan-Szechuan, Beijing, Mongolian) and pan-Asian (Southeast Asian, Korean, Japanese, and western Asia).

Some good news to report: the Eastside Community Alliance, a community cultural organization based in Oakland, California, received $7,500 from Chamber Music America to present my Afro Asian Music Ensemble sometime within the next two years. Joseph Yoon, my friend and agent, will work on putting a U.S. tour together for either fall 2007 or spring 2008.

The reading of *Dragon vs. Eagle*, a new martial arts-music/theater epic written by Ruth Margraff and I, went very well at the Apollo Theater's Salon Soundstage. The feedback and comments we received from the small group that attended both events were very helpful. It was important for us to "hear" the story performed by the seven actors and directed by Jeff Janisheski, as it gave both Ruth, myself, and producer Thaddeus Squire an opportunity to gauge the flow and clarity of the text. I was especially thrilled to be working again with an A-list group of Asian American actors in New York: Dawn Akemi Saito, Marina Celander, Perry Yung, Rick Ebihara, and Louis Ozawa Changchien. And joining them were two terrific actors whom I didn't know before: Kyle Knauf and Walker Lewis. Sometime in June 2007, the Apollo will present the full musical score performed by my Afro Asian Music Ensemble. In January 2008, we'll present a fully staged excerpt of the show with live music, martial arts choreography, lighting, costumes, and the animation.

Because I've been sleeping so much, I don't have a lot to report back to people. I want to thank Mikki Shepard, longtime friend and arts supporter, who has facilitated a discretionary grant of $2,000 to me via Thaddeus Squire's Peregrine Arts. Thank you so much for the help, as I've been unable to earn an income during my cancer war.

Chemo Session Number 9 (Only Three More to Go!)
January 25, 2007:

To my pleasant surprise, I had no allergic reaction whatsoever to the 5FU infusion. This is the first time, so my medical team has figured out the formula of premedications that work to counter the body temperature rise, the falling into unconsciousness, and the raging red rash that used to erupt. What a relief!

Perhaps because I was so happy and thrilled I didn't have any allergic reaction for the first time in the chemo treatments, even after taking a Benadryl tablet to help fall asleep, my mind was spinning with thoughts and ideas, so I really didn't fall asleep until 5:00 AM on Friday, January 26, 2007. I have to remind myself not to push myself too much. Every moment I feel good I want to do more things. But I've learning to listen to my body and my breath and to pace everything better. There are constant aggravations that I try not to let them bother or consume me, like having to be a hound dog and bill collector to get flaky people who owe me payments or the return of materials I loan them to return them to me.

I appreciate the help offered by Tina Summerlin, Melanie Dyer, Aib Gomez-Delgado, Taylor Ho Bynum, Bob Hawks, and Wolhee Choe to go to Trader Joe's and help pick up groceries. Why Trader Joe's? Because of the unique quality of their juices and other foods, the extraordinary prices, good labor practices, and wide selection, including flash frozen seafood, which is of extraordinary quality. Their juices, especially the lemon-ginger-echinacea, has had a high beneficial probiotic effect on me. Much more so than the juices I can find in your typical grocery store, bodega, or even yuppie "health" food stores.

Ruth Margraff found a wonderful 99-cent store in Astoria that sells the best natural pomegranate juice, a liter for $2.89, with very low sodium content and no additives. (A lot of highly touted juices such as noni, pomegranate, and mangosteen, have a whole bunch of additives like other cheaper juices, sugar, sodium, etc.) The juice is from Azerbaijan.

I believe the strong antioxidant juices (removing toxic free radicals) have helped to diminish the side effects of the chemo for me. The nutritional supplements and the diversity of food I've been eating have been a crucial factor in keeping my blood cell counts and chemistry very good. The plants and added oxygen exposure, along with the strong hydration, have helped with my red blood cells, which bring oxygen throughout my bloodstream, and oxygen is a strong anticancer fighter. Keeping my mind active, my soul strong, my work productive—all the result of your love and support—has kept me focused on living actively and not letting the cancer and the chemo's fatigue and sometimes very awful side effects detract, depress, or derail me from my focus.

A friend and supporter and very talented fellow warrior artist, Jen Shyu, is performing her own work this weekend. I hope all of you can go and support her. She performed wonderfully at the BAMCafé surprise event, and everyone was impressed with her and Art Hirahara and Taylor Ho Bynum.

JADE TONGUE: RITUAL
SUNDAY, JANUARY 28, 2007, 8:00 PM AND 10:00 PM
THE STONE

CORNER OF AVENUE C AND SECOND STREET, NEW YORK, NEW YORK
$10 ADMISSION, ALL PROCEEDS GO TO THE ARTISTS
JEN SHYU, VOCALS
DAVID BRYANT, PIANO
SHANE ENDSLEY, TRUMPET
BEN GERSTEIN, TROMBONE
THOMAS MORGAN, BASS
DAN WEISS, DRUMS

DIARY 10: THE FATBACK FAN CLUB

Chemo Number 10 (Only Two More Treatment Sessions to Go!)
February 6 to February 13, 2007

Chemo number 10 was relatively mild, though I was very groggy afterward and could barely keep my lids open when driving home with Earl Weathers Jr., my martial artist friend, who was kind enough to take us to Flushing, Queens, for a quick delicious lunch after the chemo.

During the treatment, we were joined by the great martial artist and teacher Sifu Gregg Zilb. Both Earl and Gregg have performed in my *Voice of the Dragon* and did the 2003 thirty-three-city U.S. tour. I enjoyed listening to their vigorous discussion about issues confronting the U.S. martial arts world, especially the controversy around mixed martial arts (MMA), which is the latest fad. Gregg is very critical of MMA as he believes it fails to teach a "system" and only eclectic trick moves and maneuvers that are ineffective for real combat. While many people may take up forms of the martial arts for differing reasons and goals (such as exercise, health, discipline, hobby, etc.), the real martial artists train for combat. The martial artists involved in the Chinese martial arts have almost all little regard for *wuxu* (the hybrid acrobatic martial arts form promoted by the Chinese government during the Cultural Revolution as an athletic competition, a kind of "gymnastics meets kung fu"), which they feel may have its merits for athletics and exercise, but ineffective for actual combat. Earl and Gregg also noted that for performance and film, *wuxu* and theatricality are important, as character expressiveness, storytelling, and dramatics are key, not combat effectiveness; however, great combat ability is still magnificent to behold, but it needs to be combined with and complement the objectives of dramatic expression for stage and film performance.

The day after the hospital chemo, I woke up very energized at 4:30 AM and started writing the speech I have to give for the Conference "What's Avant-Garde about the Avant-Garde," at the Fourth Annual

Interdisciplinary Jazz Studies Colloquium, University of Kansas. I kept writing nonstop, thoughts blazing out. I took a break midafternoon to have lunch with Peggy Choy, and Mark O'Ferrall in Flushing Chinatown, came home and started writing again. I took another break that evening to hear Derek Bermel and Wendy Walter's musical at the Flea and came home and went to bed by midnight. I didn't nap at all during the day, so it was a very long day going nonstop.

That's probably why the next day I was really, really wiped out, exhausted. I still continued to write and completed the speech, fifty-four pages long as it is the keynote address and supposed to be for an hour and a half delivery. I also didn't have much of an appetite all day. Later in the afternoon, I was able to proofread the speech and cut and edit it down some more. The speech is titled "Imagine the Impossible! Perpetuating the Avant-Garde in African American Music."

On Tuesday, our Fatback Fan Club that meets for lunch in different parts of (for now) Queens met and lunched in the Arabic section of Astoria (the northern end of Steinway Street). We had a magnificent lunch at an Egyptian place called Eastern Nights. It has a 1960s feel that could easy be a set for a Sun Ra performance, with an orange-lighted backroom-outdoor patio area. The week before, we had lunch at a Moroccan eatery in the same area. The two block area is lined with hookah (water pipe) lounges along with restaurants and grocery stores. The best pita bread, completely free of chemical preservatives and additives, is a brand called Pita Express made on Utica Avenue in Brooklyn, found in one of the Astoria local small grocery stores where you can also buy Arabic music and musical instruments!

As I prepare to finish my chemo treatments (number 11 and number 12 and then I'm done!), I want to share the lessons and transformations I've learned and experienced.

WHAT I HAVE LEARNED

First, the love and support of family and friends have been the key advantage I have in the cancer war. Without allies and broad support, no war is winnable (witness the U.S. situation today in Iraq and Afghanistan). All of you have contributed in a special synergy that many people, sadly, lack in their support. Because of the diverse, eclectic, and broad types of people in my life, all of whom are of high integrity, responsibility, intelligence, and capability in your own right, I have a proactive community. The fact that Sgt. Major Magdalena Gómez and General Ann T. Greene organized our LISTSERV community, marshaled the forces, distributed and scheduled assignments, etc., relieved tremendous stress, worries, and logistical details from me. I could concentrate on key matters such as fighting my HMO, learning to fight on a cellular level (see below), and daily health matters. Even when I was dealing with the problem of insurance, etc., friends with legal expertise and contacts offered lawyer contacts, etc. People brought over delicious and nutritious foods, offered their cars to drive me to appointments, or simply go out and have a normal life. People's gifts, donations, well wishes, cards, e-mails, phone calls, etc., never made me feel alone, isolated, depressed, or hopeless. Gwen Mok and others rallied to fight the Frigidaire-Electrolux corporation and got me a brand-new refrigerator. People who accompanied me to my chemo sessions gave me support during a harrowing time. The very first treatment of the 5FU drug produced a terrible allergic reaction that sent the nurses and physician's assistant into alarm mode, but having my friend Ruth Margraff there gave me a sense of confidence that should something disastrous happen, a trusted friend would be a witness. Luckily, nothing did.

On the medical front, having such intelligent and capable friends put all the medical staff on notice. They knew that a circle of very smart and proactive people surrounded me, who wouldn't let anything slide. My sister Florence is a doctor and administrator at the U.S. FDA and spoke to my gastroenterologist, my surgeon, and my oncologist. So all the professionals responsible for my care and treatment knew that knowledgeable, expert, and caring people all followed my situation. Indeed, after my surgery and recovery, I sent a complimentary letter about certain staff people, which greatly helped their careers. I also sent a critical evaluation of certain staff who were incompetent, uncaring, and unresponsive. At least one of these persons was fired.

Second, I quickly learned that I, the patient, must take charge of my own improvement and recovery. Too many people just think, my doctors are the professionals, it's their job to fix me and do very little or nothing to improve themselves. That's the overreliance on medical science, the assumption that technology and science are the cure-all and total fix-it.

Third, learning to fight on the cellular level involves three key areas: *hydration, oxygenation, and nutrition.* The human body is 70 percent water with an array of other elements, minerals, etc. I believe that drinking a vast diversity of probiotic liquids supported and stimulated healthy cell production and sustenance. Liquids to avoid completely are coffee and caffeinated beverages, anything loaded with sweeteners and alcohol. Liquids to drink are 100 percent juices or, better, fresh-squeezed; a wide assortment of teas; and mineral water. Cancer cells thrive on antioxygenation, suffocating and preventing oxygen. Regular deep-breathing exercises, surrounding oneself with oxygen-producing plants, having a high antioxidant diet that removes harmful and toxic free radicals, all are positive. You have to eat to live, but what you eat must be life enhancing, not life debilitating. My strong blood cell counts, my low incidence of nausea and diarrhea, and my very good chemistry results I attribute to the attention paid to nutrition, using daily multivitamin supplements, selenium (antitumor fighter), ginseng, green magma, 1000 mg daily of vitamin C, etc.

Bob Lederer especially convinced me of the importance of high-quality multivitamin supplements (www.supernutritionusa.com) from his activism in the anti-AIDS war. Limor Tomer convinced me that the overall degradation of our food has made it necessary that we bolster our nutrition with strong, quality supplements. In combining the three areas of hydration, oxygenation, and nutrition, I have changed my diet toward far greater sources of raw foods, including fruits and vegetables and sashimi (raw fish). Overcooking at high heats kills the nutritional content of food. Raw is best, then steamed or quick-blanched, then baked or quickly stir-fried. Grilling, deep-frying, and broiling are the worst. I can actually now feel now my body reacts. My body braces against high-heat cooking and is relaxed with raw or low-heat cooked foods. A good and delicious way to consume raw fruits and vegetables is fresh-squeezing them into juices. Any part of food that is "burned" is potentially carcinogenic. Just as breathing or eating anything smoked. Hydration, oxygenation, and nutrition are eliminated by high heat.

Fourth, fortifying the mental, emotional, and spiritual. Every day in war has pain and suffering. That is why we should and must avoid wars of all kinds unless they become absolutely necessary (to save our lives, including saving the planet which sustains human life). If those who made the decisions to go to war actually themselves had to experience direct pain and suffering, such decisions would not be easily or readily made. There is extreme volatility (very bad and very good days) to a general malaise and trauma (constant fatigue, weariness, exhaustion). It is important to *never* allow oneself to have doubt, depression, despair. All my great circle of friends never allowed me to feel isolated, letting me know that I could call on someone for help of any kind, or that people would regularly come and visit and talk with me.

I listened a lot to music of all kinds, but the best was the least-"processed" music. The Jajouka music of the Gnawa people from the Atlas Mountain of Morocco (CD-RS given to me by Kim Tinsley), Hawaiian music (given to me by Richard Hamasaki and Marina Celander), and my vast collection of Korean folk music and folk opera (*pansori*), and of course the free jazz of the U.S. 1960s–1970s (what I prefer to call "the vanguard music of the Black Arts Movement") all helped to lift my spirits, move my body, fire my soul and imagination. Even when I was too exhausted to practice my sax or compose music, just by listening to music, or in mind, figuring out complex rhythms in "odd" meters (just as 7/8 or 9/8 or 11/8 or 13/8 or 15/8 or 17/8) were challenges to me, but also provided new discoveries that gave me excitement from the joy of investigation, practice, and application (finally figuring them out).

The next journal will share with you in-depth my thoughts about how fighting cancer has changed me.

Big thanks to Diane Fujino and her family for sending a gift of $250.

DIARY 11: CHEMO NUMBER 11 (ONE MORE TO GO!)

February 22, 2007

In Memoriam: LeRoy Jenkins, the great violinist-improviser-composer, passed away on February 24, 2007, from lung cancer at the age of *seventy-four*. A major figure in the new jazz (or vanguard music of the Black Arts Movement) since the 1960s, I last heard LeRoy perform one the most incredible free improvised solos at Roulette a couple of years ago when the Brooklyn Sax Quartet shared the evening with him. During the 1980s, LeRoy performed in my *Cal Massey Tribute Orchestra* project, having himself been a former member of the legendary RoMas Orchestra co-led by Cal and Italian American socialist composer-arranger Romulus Franceschini from the 1960s to Cal's death in the early 1970s. We miss LeRoy and his music. Thank you to Weihua Zhang for her donation of $100.

What do you say to the following?

After surgery for breast cancer at Memorial Sloan-Kettering, the most well-funded, prestigious cancer research and treatment center in the United States, many patients immediately after surgery go outside to smoke their cigarettes.

Or even more ironic, how such an institution will only accept two insurance plans: Blue Cross-Blue Shield (one of the most expensive plans) or Medicaid (very tough to qualify for if you aren't completely indigent, homeless, unable to leave your domicile, unable to speak English or not of Native American certified ethnicity). Basically the latter is accepted so as to not be completely "transparent" for being classist as an institution that prefers the affluent patient.

Or after billions of dollars spent for decades on finding a cure for cancer, that virtually no progress has been made, the number of cancer patients has grown (though for some cancers, such as colon cancer, figures seem to be dropping; and cervical cancer seems to have found a vaccine), more and perhaps better treatments have been developed and implemented, but well over a million people die annually? After vehicular homicide, cancer is the second-largest killer of Americans.

Or knowing other cancer patients at stage 4 (terminal) who are twenty-seven years old, suffering from lung or breast cancer even though they never smoked a cigarette in their life but lived with parents who smoked like chimneys and probably got their cancer through secondhand smoke exposure. The parents continue to smoke, even in the presence of their daughter who is at stage four. And this twenty-seven-year-old is engaged to be married, knowing full well that the number of years or perhaps months that she has to live is very uncertain.

I am someone who believes in the struggle to find answers. Cataloging or observing the effects of problems isn't enough for me. I have to know *why*. And as poet Amiri Baraka poetically intones, knowing the whys makes us wise. Once we truly understand *why* can be begin to change the root causes of the effects, conditions, and symptoms, to do something real and substantive, which always begins first by changing ourselves, our thinking about the problem(s), and our behavior and course of action.

I have fundamentally changed my life several times during the course of my adult life. There have been several paradigm shifts (what Thomas Kuhn termed for major "scientific revolutions" in Western science). I don't believe in stasis: we are all constantly changing, even at the cellular level. The question is, How are we changing, and is it for the better?

Here is how I have changed most recently in the war against cancer:

First, while I still retain my iron discipline, broad outlook and openness, antiprocrastination and ability to multitask, and move decisively, I have accepted that the purpose must and should not be for egotistical competitiveness, career aggrandizement, accumulation of the quantitative, or for approval, acceptance, and reward from the mainstream status quo. Rather, self-development should be its own standard that is oftentimes counter to status quo terms and conceptions of success. I more than ever realize the value and importance of my friendships with all the fellow warriors who have been part of this LISTSERV and the many others who have expressed sympathy and given support to me in the war against cancer, that, as Magdalena Gómez expressed it, the point of setting standards and striving for integrity and excellence is to evoke the transformation and transcendence of those around you, to inspire one another as part of enhancing all of our contributions to transform society and the world to be free of exploitation, injustice, inequality, and oppression.

Second, in accepting Ludditism (*Contrary to popular mythology, the Luddites did not oppose machines per se, but "machinery hurtful to Commonality"—Mitchel Cohen*), I have come to reject technological-industrial fetishism (both meanings of fetish—the traditional meaning of conferring power to something and the Freudian concept of obsession with something). Industrial organization and the over-reliance of technology as a fix-it-all solution intrinsically contains the destructive and exploitative content of the capitalist system that engendered and shaped its development and character. Therefore, that which is bigger, faster, more efficient, more powerful is *not* necessarily better and in the terms and manifestations of capitalism, often toxic, destructive and inimical to commonality (the well-being of the ecological systems and organisms of the planet, including the social ones necessary to humanity). Cancer cannot and will not be cured as long as there is more profit (money to be made) in "managing" it, in coming up with newer and more expensive "power drugs and treatments" rather than eliminating pesticides, environmental toxicity, greatly reducing processed foods and chemical additives, prepared food businesses that rely upon deep-fried and high-temperature/burned cooking, the cigarette industry, a privatized profiteering insurance company multipayer industry instead of a single-payer national health insurance system, etc.

Third, I have clearly decided to get off the treadmill of accumulation or what is also called the rat race. How much money is enough? How much do you really need? What is the price for peace, satisfaction, happiness, health, and creativity? I found something very interesting said by President Fidel Castro of Cuba. One unexpected environmentalist posed this question to Castro: "Should we expect that densely populated countries, such as China, India, Indonesia, will have as many automobiles in proportion to their population as North America and Western Europe?" Castro answered, "Well, it's necessary; the expansion of capital requires it. It's also impossible; the earth cannot sustain it."

In 2000, I sold my former duplex loft in yuppie Park Slope, and I also sold 70 percent of my material belongings, keeping only four pieces of furniture: a $30 dining table my mother bought for me thirty years ago, a four-drawer wood file cabinet I bought in 1977 for $35, a bookshelf/file cabinet I bought at a secondhand office furniture store on Canal Street, and a pullout futon sofa couch for $100 in the early 1990s. Most of what I kept were my books and LPs (bought mostly secondhand over many years) and the clothes I've been designing for myself since 1989, along with kitchenware. Contrary to most Americans, I did not buy a bigger place, but I downsized my life entirely. I simplified it as well, knowing that I would probably not ever get married or raise children. I did *not* go into greater debt, decided to divest myself of much material belongings, and decided that the most important accumulations would be *experiences* (whatever, wherever, whenever). I vowed that if I could live in NYC on $15,000 a year, comfortably, then I would be on a new path to freedom, peace, satisfaction, happiness, health, and creativity by *never* having to compromise for money. I believe my cancer started about ten years ago (my sister dates that based on the size of my tumor and the medical data she has studied working for the FDA in cancer pharmaceuticals) when I was living in the duplex loft in Park Slope on the treadmill of pursuing a competitively aggressive career. Though I was never blinded or obsessed with this, as I continued to be a very dedicated and committed radical activist during that time as well, I nonetheless began to take on the lifestyle of a yuppie artist living in Park Slope. Yes, I had joined the Park Slope Food Coop to both eat healthier and to support socially progressive food politics; nonetheless, what was my daily diet? Broiled steak, a salad with high-fat dressing over steamed white rice, drinking milkshakes, microwaving leftovers, barbequing on my roof smoked and burnt chicken, beef, some tofu and grilled veggies, getting a big lunch plate of MSG-saturated yellow rice, high-sodium cooked beans, and broiled, roasted, or grilled meats.

After selling the loft for a handsome profit, refusing to buy a bigger place and incur debt, I bought a much smaller place for a fraction of what I made from the sale of the loft, designed the place myself, and am much happier, peaceful, satisfied than before. Add to that the monetary success I had from the *Voice of the Dragon* tour, I have enough money for the rest of my life if I stay at the $15,000 a year personal budget. I work *not* for money anymore, but to work with the artists I want to work with on the projects I want to do (the criteria for which is simple: projects that *no one* else would ever do because they don't fit). Given the life-threatening nature of cancer, I have constructed a will that upon my death all my assets be sold in order to finance the Fred Ho Foundation, which will have the simple and sole mission of giving direct funding annually to a worthy radical and transgressive artist to be spent at his/her discretion.

Fourth, I have come to appreciate, recognize, and learn the power of one's breath. To breathe deeply daily and to *listen* to one's breath is to feel and "hear" one's soul. Some practice meditation or *chi-gong*. The common purpose is to take time from daily business and busy-ness to simply be elemental, to oxygenate oneself, to take a "breathe-er," to appreciate another day alive on this planet. Many have wondered and asked me how has my saxophone playing been in all this since I am often very fatigued, didn't practice for five weeks recovering from surgery (and declined performing at the Guggenheim concerts with singer Haleh Abghari since my diaphragm hadn't healed), and cancelled all my performing engagements during postsurgery and chemotherapy treatments for six months. Well, let me tell you that I believe my saxophone playing and my musical consciousness have attained a level of transcendence I could not previously expect nor imagine. I wrote this to composer-friend Stefan Hakenberg when he asked me via e-mail how has my saxophone playing been in this cancer war:

My sax playing is very strong, even stronger than before I entered surgery. After surgery, my diaphragm had to heal before I could play again. But now I play with a lot more power and control. This stems from the breathing exercises I've been doing, but also from the development of my chi energy. I basically have outgrown everything made for the bari sax. There isn't a big-enough mouthpiece commercially made for me. I need reeds harder/ stronger than the number 5, the hardest commercially made. I play the horn now like a double-reed instrument, barely touching the reed with my embouchure. From the power of my breath along, I can make it vibrate without touching it. My fingers have molded the ivory and brass to fit my hands. I have actually altered metal from years of my touch. It is truly man over metal. I have also discovered some very Daoist revelations:

The point of developing technique is to have *no* technique;

The point of practicing and mastery is to develop chi so that music can change the world (both social and natural);

I want my sound to bring down the walls of Jericho, to be a biblical-like force to crush the walls of poverty, exploitation, and oppression;

I want to be as a soloist more powerfully expressive and convicted than a seventy-piece professional orchestra; and to improvise as great as a sophisticated, complex, notated score;

I want to have a band that is telepathic, taking what is notated on the written page to a higher level of expression beyond what even I as the composer-leader could ever imagine.

The war against cancer has brought about this transformation, revelation, and application on my part. I have been tremendously humbled by this war and at the same time learned to fight on a cellular level and to apply a cellular approach to the technical, emotional, creative, and spiritual challenges of making music. The cells of one's sound is what is supreme, infusing one's breath or chi energy to that cellular vibration of making one's sound a life-force.

Fifth, and probably the *most* important transformation for me: to never harbor envy, jealously, competitiveness, to speak the truth (even if it is very critical of friends and loved ones, but to do so without comparison and always with compassion), to know that should I die soon, I will be happy and satisfied with what I've done, and to spend not an iota of energy of mine worrying or despondent about my condition (though to take it seriously and fight with all my being to win the war against cancer), but to devote my energy both in my personal war against cancer, but as a friend to all of you, to make us all better in our journeys as emotional, creative, and intellectual beings on this planet.

The death of cancer will only come about when the very conditions of toxicity that give growth to cancer cells have been eliminated. What we are faced with is how systemic the conditions of toxicity are: engendered and enhanced by all the things that are accepted as natural to capitalist-industrial society (sadly, imitated and not thoroughly challenged or countered by many socialist societies, both present and collapsed). The constantly expanding exposure to many forms of electromagnetic radiation, the shredding of the natural ozone layer that protects us from the sun's harmful UVA and UVB radiation, the pollutant poisons we dump into the air, earth, and bodies of water, the fluorocarbons emitted by refrigerators and carbon-burning cars, the saturation of chemicals in our food, the nutritional degradation of our food, the toxin chemicals that permeate our dry cleaning, shampoos, etc., our overall weakened immune system from nutritional deficiency, over-reliance on chemical vaccines and treatments, and the list goes on and on and on because all these are manifestations of modern, industrial capitalist existence. It is more profitable to manage than to cure/solve. The one basic fundamental of capitalism is this: it is a system that has created the power to feed, clothe, house everyone, and to remake or destroy the world; but at the heart of it all, it is a system that creates more problems than it solves.

While my philosophical-political worldview remains what it was prior to getting cancer, the war has taught me important lessons and changed me in profound ways that may never have happened if I didn't have to face it myself. It is the experience of fighting cancer that has instilled a new imagination in me about how to fight to detoxify and liberate ourselves and the world

My final cancer war diary journal entry will come around March 10, 2007. I hope that there will not be a recurrence that will require another war journal. The war will continue for a long time, not only for me personally to make sure no cancer cells ever grow again inside of me, but to support the ongoing greater war to remove the cancer of capitalism from this world.

DIARY 12: THE CELLS OF ONE'S SOUND—CHEMO NUMBER 12 (THE FINAL TREATMENT)

March 22, 2007

Thank you to Bill V. Mullen of the American Studies Department at Purdue University in Indiana for bringing poet Magdalena Gómez and me (on baritone sax) to perform on March 2, 2007. It was my first public performance since being diagnosed with cancer on August 4, 2006. Even though with airport delays to and from, I had sufficient energy to perform at a level that met my satisfaction, though I did sleep for ten hours afterward! We all enjoyed meeting Bill's fiancée Tithi, a joyous and smart professor of South Asian History at Purdue. They will get married in India in June of this year. It was also nice seeing Bill's teenage son, Max. Bill and I have collaborated on a massive anthology titled *Afro Asia: Revolutionary Political and Cultural Connections between African- and Asian-Americas* to be published by Duke University Press.

This is my last cancer war journal entry unless the war starts up again and cancer returns and I fail to make it into remission. But read below about this.

On March 8, I woke up at 5:40 AM to get ready for the Access-A-Ride van that came at 6:25 AM to take me to my final chemo treatment at the Ambulatory Chemo Treatment (ACT) Center of the Long Island Jewish Medical Center. I always dread these sessions because of the previous allergic reactions, the extreme drowsiness brought on by the Benadryl medication, and the thought of thousands of milligrams of toxic chemicals saturating me. Perhaps this anxiety might explain the higher blood pressure readings I get there: at the start of the day 150/110 (very bad) and at the end of the day 140/97 (lower but still bad). But then when I'm home and the visiting nurse takes my blood pressure, such as this evening (and she did it twice to be sure), it was 120/70 (very good). As the chemo phase of my treatment and recovery has ended, part of the next phase of my recovery and rebuilding will be to nail my blood pressure to no higher than 120/80 and to lose twenty pounds from intensive cardio training (butterfly swimming and crawl and breast stroke sprinting, instead of the stamina and distance focus I had before cancer of swimming a mile in one hour).

I have changed my priorities significantly. These are my new priorities in life: swimming, exercise, walking at least half an hour daily, eating for pleasure but with nutrition as the core of that pleasure, enjoying my friends and family, and taking on projects that *no one* else would touch that have no mainstream appeal, interest or support, but which need to confront and challenge and change the consciousness of people.

I have lost all interest in pursuing a career. Even before cancer, I had the mentality that if it felt like I was working on a career, then I should stop, get over it, and let someone who can do it better and kick my ass to have the spotlight without me being their competitor. Today, the pursuit of money isn't important except in issues of furthering fairness, justice, and making sure I can adequately and justly compensate the talented people who work on my projects. A long time ago, I told a girlfriend who wanted to discuss marriage and raising a family with me, "If it came to a choice of paying my artists or feeding my kids, my kids would starve." Her reply, "Good thing you don't have kids." I was clear then that monogamy, marriage, and the nuclear family weren't going to work for me.

Anything that implies or complies with material accumulation and accumulation for me will be resisted with all my might. I have *everything I need and want in life*, and if I die today, I'd be satisfied with what I've contributed and created as templates, precursors, exemplars, and experiments for a new society. A lot more needs to be done, and every day I have more to live, will be devoted to figuring out by example and experimentation on *how* to make the impossible. Sun Ra said something that strikes at the necessity of uniting imagination and revolution: "Everything possible has been done and nothing has changed. What we need is the impossible." *Yes*: impossible ideas and activities.

And something else I've come to understand: "Vision and imagination without discipline is dreaming. Discipline without vision and imagination is brutality."

I have been prepared for death a long time ago, since from a very young, early age. And once I accepted it, I lost all fear of it. I have accepted that I could be murdered, die of accidents (several were very close, which I will briefly describe below), and now, die from illness. I can't forecast whatever form of death there is since those three categories seem to encompass all the possibilities, but maybe there might be other forms of death we haven't conceived. Of course, yes, suicide. But I eliminated self-destruction a very long time ago. I wholly support euthanasia and would do it myself rather than know that I would live without the ability to control my own destiny or be able to fight anymore. I would ask all my friends to support that decision and possibly assist me if your conscience would allow it.

It is this acceptance of death and the lack of fear that enabled me to become a warrior because I could be decisive without any reservations, doubts, fears, anxieties, and uncertainties about my commitment to take on whatever challenges and new chapters in my life that I would embark upon.

I never regretted or dwelled upon the tens of thousands of dollars of money I've risked and lost on personal and professional projects.

Or be in shock or fear when the car I was in with two other people hit an icy patch on a highway and the car did a 180-degree flip and jumped the guard rail and landed on the opposite lane against traffic. Luckily no one was injured, and we weren't crushed or hit by oncoming traffic.

Or worry when massive waves and rip currents during the many times I've been snorkeling in extremely dangerous snorkeling situations would hurl me like a leaf in the ocean and I had to accept fate and my understanding of currents to know that eventually everything gets sent to shore.

Or face racist marines wanting to street fight me.

Or be trapped in a whale ring with three sixty-foot-long humpback whales heading straight toward our two-man sea kayak in the Admiralty Straights of Alaska. I trusted that the whales, masters of their denizen, were in control of everything and, though "wild" animals, would "decide" our fate, and we wouldn't have any control over it.

Or have snarling parental sea lions in shark-infested waters in the Channel Islands, wondering if they would allow me to stay my distance while I observed their frolicking precious young cubs. I always carry a knife with me while snorkeling. I would fight any creature (including humans) that attacked me, though I first would do the cardinal rule of self-defense: stay out of harm's way and turn away from conflict. If that conflict, however, is brought onto me, then the only decision is to fight to win. I never could be a pacifist.

And the fight against cancer is my most recent war saga. But it is very hopeful. In fact, my medical team today described my situation as "amazing" (their descriptor). The physician assistant (PA) said that the staff hadn't seen anyone like me whose chemistry and blood counts have consistently stayed strong and that I never required any medication to boost them from danger levels or from consistent downward trends. The CEA test (carcinogenic embryonic antigen) for detecting the presence and increase/decrease of cancer cells has remained a flat line at zero from October to the end of December 2006, very positive and encouraging. They didn't know that I had learned to fight on a cellular level. They just concluded, "You are a very strong person."

The usual symptoms of shriveling up, loss of hair, weight loss, terrible nausea, constant diarrhea, projectile vomiting, severe peripheral neuropathy (loss of manual dexterity and inability to tell if my fingers or toes and feet were moving at all), swelling of the ankles, severe infections from my mouth to my anus, contracting viral infections, failure to clot from cuts, skin breakage, gum and mouth sores, etc., I never had. Yes, constant fatigue (from the accumulation and saturation of tremendous amounts of toxic chemo drugs since I get the biggest dosage since I have very large body mass); yes, some diarrhea and nausea in the early treatments; and yes, constant peripheral neuropathy, which is the sensation of my fingers and toes feeling they are frostbitten all the time, but not any loss of dexterity since I can type this journal and handwrite music and play the sax. Hopefully, in most cases, these symptoms disappear in time, anywhere from weeks to months to over a year. Some symptoms may remain for life, and they are highly individual specific. For example, my youngest sister who has successfully fought cervical cancer can't eat spicy foods anymore. I find I'm preferring a raw-food diet more and more. Even turkey burgers, while I can have psychosympathetic cravings for them, once I made them and started eating, I didn't really enjoy them. I must confess that from time to time I really do miss the taste of beef, especially hamburgers and shell, T-bone, and rib eye steaks.

After the first four treatments, I stopped using the antinausea and antidiarrhea medication that were prescribed to me. Today, I donated them to the ACT center, and the PA was very happy to get them as some patients' insurances won't pay for these expensive pills that cost as much as $60 a pill!

Even before cancer, I was determined to live as much of a chemical-free life as I possibly could. But as you read in my journals, I don't subscribe to relying on alternative medicine and treatments. The data and studies haven't supported anything hopeful upon a regimen that solely is based on alternative approaches. I believe they can be useful and important supplements (e.g., taking selenium as an antitumor fighter or certain Chinese herbs or using ginseng). But the evidence is that if I didn't do the FOLFOX chemo regimen, I would have only a 20 percent chance of survival. Of course, you can always find in the homeopathic literature and hype a lot of anecdotal and observational examples marveling at certain individual recoveries and even miraculous cures. That might be the case, but without statistical studies, they are like lottery stories. People who play the lottery can win tens, hundreds, thousands, ten thousands, and even millions of dollars; but even those lucky winners' stories are fraught with government tax problems, inability to deal with financial management issues, family dissensions and havoc, and many other problems that aren't given attention in the media.

And mainstream medical science, as I've discussed in other war journals, are also fraught with many problems stemming from the structural imperatives and designs of a capitalist health care industry that favors profits and precludes the primacy of patients and the necessary social and environmental solutions.

What's next?

I will continue to have monthly blood and chemistry tests every six months; according to the clinical trial protocols I've obligated to, I must have a CT scan and an annual colonoscopy. Early detection of recurring cancer cell growth will be the key to how the next war will be fought, should there be a next war, which we all hope there won't be. But I have realized that I can't rely upon the doctors and experts to be the sole power. I must make the transformations to heighten my abilities as an anticancer, anticapitalist, prosocialist/communist, pro-Luddite, promatriarchalist warrior. I discussed above my new priorities. Fellow cancer warrior Michael Surdei reached out to me upon the recommendation of Magdalena Gómez. Without knowing me, but given the imprimatur by Magdalena, he has become a good buddy, bringing me plants for oxygenation, taking me out to our Fatback Fan Club lunches, holding forth with his stories, being a militant and didactic lecturer about what I "should" consider, and always offering assistance in actions to solve my problems. I have more opened myself to old and new friends and the marvels they bring to my life, which has sustained my spirit. Old wounds and "issues" have been healed and discarded. It is easier now to apologize, to not hold on and to see the good that can still be increased, and the friendship that can move on to a new level of understanding and sharing.

Derek Bermel, Jen Shyu, Ashley Baylor and Stephen Jackson, Quincy and Margaret Troupe, Gladys Serrano, Peter Adelman and Paget Walker, Yumi Kurosawa, Rick Ebihara, the best sushi in NYC brought over by Shanmin Yu, Shoba Narayana, Abraham Gomez-Delgado and Ayesha, Steve Carlino, David Bindman, David Kastin, Bob Lederer and John Riley, the noni Juices from Yoshi Amao, Richard Hamasaki and Mika Saburi, Peggy Choy, Marina Celander and her family, the Greene-O'Ferrall clan, my sisters Flora and Florence, Taylor Ho Bynum, John Duffy's juices from Maine, Wolhee Choe and Bob Hawks, Deb Gilbert and Scott Kegelsmann, and others, all made time and effort to come over, bringing food, and groceries.

Many others like Mary Sharp Cronson, Baraka Sele, Jayne Cortez, John Duffy, Mikki Shepard, Salim Washington and Melanie Dyer (who contributed groceries from my favorite Trader Joe's), Weihua Zhang, Frances Goldin, Idell Conaway, the Fujino-Harmacchus family, the folks at the Brooklyn Academy of Music, and all the artists who performed at my tribute and donated their artists fees, gave generous financial donations that helped me buy food and groceries, pay bills, etc. Others sent music, cards, poetry, teas, organic fruits and juices (Samantha Smart, Claire Milardi, Thomas Buckner, and Kamala Cesar), writings, prayers, thoughts, and loving well wishes. All those who drove and accompanied me to chemo treatments, getting up early in the morning and observing me connected to chemo infusions, or people who simply made themselves to be chauffeurs and helpers: Earl Weathers Jr., Gregg Zilb, Jon Ogilvy (with support from Catherine Patterson), Bob and Wolhee Choe, Ruth Margraff, Jen Feil, Paget Walker, Derek Bermel, Cristian Amigo, Taylor Ho Bynum and Gwen

Mok and Peggy Choy, Jim Fleming, Deb Gilbert, Mike Surdei, Art Hirahara, Tina Summerlin, Mark O'Ferrall, Daystarr and Evergreen Chou, Thaddeus Squire, and others.

The Japan Society Performing Arts Division and the Civitella Raineri Foundation graciously gave me flowers and a membership to the Brooklyn Botanical Garden for oxygenation.

And of course, my great medical team: Dr. Edith Mitchell whose second opinions were invaluable and the help given to me by oncology nurse Vicki Squire to investigate clinical trials and to arrange the consultation with Dr. Mitchell; Dr. Chao Chen, my primary care physician; Dr. Richard Emmanuel, gastroenterologist who performed my colonoscopy; Dr. Evan Berman, my surgeon-extraordinaire; Dr. Kalaria, who implanted my Medi-port; the nursing staff during my surgery, especially Richard Miller, Anschel Hyacinthe, and others; Dr. Dilip Patel, my primary oncologist and his caring and professionally excellent staff of physicians, researchers, physician assistants, registered nurses, and oncology nurses. There were leading physicians and team support staff in all phases of my war: from diagnosis, to surgery, to chemo treatment. A lot of information and navigation and difficult decisions had to be made in a very short amount of time given the urgency of my staging at 3b (from size of tumor, spread into intestinal tissue, presence of carcinoma in lymph nodes). Important and invaluable help came from my sister Florence, an FDA administrator and specialist in cancer pharmaceuticals, as well as my other sister Flora, who fought cervix cancer twice and had tremendous experiences she shared with me in preparation for what I would confront. My sister-warrior!

I must praise again the leading roles of General Ann T. Greene for initially marshalling the troops and organizing the assignments and joining Sgt. Major Magdalena Gomez (or should I classify them as "high priestesses" per Peggy Choy's opinion) to erect the LISTSERV Warriors for Fred, and along with Jen Feil and Paget Walker and Peter Adelman saw me through the surgery period when I could barely walk and was most dependent upon people to cook and do chores. They came through hitting the ground hard and running. Magdalena even took three weeks off to live with me to make sure I was cared for, with detriment to her health and finances. This is a love supreme.

All the friends from afar who called, wrote, and e-mailed me from Hawaii, to Arizona, to California, to Europe, to Japan, to Taiwan and Thailand, to Trinidad and Latin America. Old friends like Jesse Wardlow, Bill Fletcher, Roy Smith, Felipe Noguera, Sarah Dupuy, Jill Ives, Ricardo Gomes, Hafez Modirzadeh—so many . . .

And there is the Mellow Warrior, the greatest love of my life, my soul mate.

The self-organization, initiative, generosity, and consistency of all my friends, simply shows that we are the cells (take it however you want to politically or metaphorically!) for a future humanity of self-governing collectively autonomous producers (i.e., people who get things done, whose walk is always greater than their talk, though whose talk is highly poetical and fabulous as well!).

I will take things a lot slower than I did with my previous alpha personality. And I hope all of you will respect and appreciate this. I will always honor everyone who reaches out to me and return your e-mails, phone calls, letters, anything, within forty-eight hours. I will never be flaky. I might never become the darling of anyone in the establishment and never get the budgets most who have attained some degree of establishment favor or support, however partial or temporary. Continuing as a guerrilla outsider is what I've been, and I'm prepared to be this for the rest of my stay on this planet, or until I decide to exit modern civilization should my cancer recur (remember, I made this vow in an early cancer war journal).

I have decided to be as self-reliant and independent of the mainstream as I can be and only work with those in the mainstream (such as certain presenters and curators) that can easily—without evasion, deflection, avoidance and run-arounds—make a commitment to work with me and carry it out with decisiveness, integrity, commitment to professional excellence, and boldness: the very same qualities I work with. Career doesn't matter to me. In fact, I have struggling to eliminate it from my consciousness. In my personal life and psyche, I have everything I need and want. I don't want to accumulate or consume more in terms of material things. Indeed, as I've shared my perspective with all of you, I believe that the world cannot sustain the American standard of living, let alone the fetishism of technology should that standard of living be projected as a standard for the rest of the world. Indeed, part of the revolution will be for first worlders to accept a decrease in wealth and affluence as part of redistribution and reallocation of resources, but also as part of dramatically reducing waste and consumption greatly harmful to the planet's ecology. Men will have to accept matriarchy as part of the overthrow of patriarchy, the redistribution and reallocation of power and control. We will win the war on cancer when we eliminate pesticides, the environmental toxicity of industrialism and mass production and waste, and change food production and consumption towards organic, nutrition-enhancing, probiotic, diversified, and localized modes, and construct single-payer socialized medicine that integrates allopathic and alternative approaches along with a paradigm shift that unites science with revolutionary social change.

Let us work together because that is what our soul tells us and find the resources we need, albeit minimal, but still make magic because we are truly creative and imaginative. Our word, discipline, and unique exemplary capabilities, respect and honoring of each other, as well as the fun we have and the love for another shall be our power.

This journal ends here, but our journey together continues. . .

THE WARRIORS FOR FRED LISTSERV IS NOW REACTIVATED

On September 24, 2007, a tumor was found again almost in the same location in my colon as found during my first colonoscopy when the original cancer diagnosis happened on August 4, 2006. The war against colon cancer continues. Surgery (again) will have to be performed as soon as possible.

In round 1 of the war against cancer, all of you gave me such tremendous and invaluable love, support/assistance, and friendship, which has essentially kept me alive. I am forever grateful. I will continue to need your love, assistance, and friendship in this new round of the war.

HERE IS MY CURRENT STATUS AS OF SEPTEMBER 26, 2007

A small tumor (about 2 to 2.5 centimeters) exists at the point of resectioning of my colon from the surgery that happened August 25, 2006. My oncologist, Dr. Dilip Patel, has ordered CT and PET scans to check on any spread to vital organs such as my kidney and liver. Those tests will be done sometime in the next two to three weeks. All my blood tests are excellent, giving hope that perhaps the cancer is localized. If it is local, I may only need surgery. If it isn't then and has spread to vital organs, then surgery isn't possible to those organs and new treatments (chemo? radiation?) will be necessary. The objective presently is to see if there is any indication of spread. *We are also preparing for surgery to remove the tumor, which should happen around the end of October/early November.*

HOW YOU CAN HELP

I will need time to rest and recover from the surgery and receiving a lot of phone calls will disturb that. Visits are best arranged via e-mail as well, so please list specific date and time options.

Based on the last battle, one of the ongoing needs is driving transportation. For those who have cars available during the day and can drive, please contact Ann T. Greene.

There were many lessons learned from the last battle. My surgery will occur soon (exact date will be forthcoming); I will remain for five to seven days in the hospital and then return home. At home, I will be unable to do much for the first three weeks, unable to lift or carry anything, and struggling to walk and sit upright again. If you recall, walking one block was a real effort. Here is what I am asking for if you can help:

1. *To borrow a personal CD player with headphones* while I am in the hospital. This allowed me to hear the healing power of music and to zone out from the mayhem in the hospital.
2. A negligent nurse last time almost killed me by shutting off my drainage tubing while I slept. Luckily the surgeon came in early the next morning and found this situation and frantically fixed it. *I would like companionship to sleep overnight in my hospital room for the first three nights I am in the hospital.*
3. *Visiting me at the hospital brings me great joy, as well as visiting me at home*, helping me take a daily walk around the block.
4. I will need *help shopping for groceries and other physical labor assistance* that I will be unable to perform.
5. *I ask that you refrain from calling me on the phone; the best thing is to contact Ann to schedule a visit* to come over to my place. Ann can e-mail you directions to my place and let you know what you could possibly bring or how you may possibly help.

Finally, I hope all of you can make my last concert before I have surgery:

My last performance for a while will be the twenty-fifth anniversary celebration of my band, the Afro Asian Music Ensemble. It would mean a lot to me if you all could come. Please call and make your reservations as soon as you can.

Fred Ho and the Afro Asian Music Ensemble celebrate their twenty-fifth anniversary in what is expected to be an extraordinary concert on Thursday, October 25, 2007 at 8:30 PM, Ninety-sixth Street west of Broadway (enter side entrance to Symphony Space).

Opening the concert will be the NYC premiere of Fred Ho's "Suite for Matriarchal Shaman Warriors" performed by an amazing group, IIIZ+ (Japanese *koto*, Korean kumungo, Chinese guzheng, and Korean percussion). The second half will feature the Fred Ho's score to "The Deadly She-Wolf Assassin at Armageddon"!

A FAR ROUGHER WAR—A SECOND TUMOR IS FOUND

On November 14, 2007, after a whole new series of tests including a second colonoscopy (October 30), CT/PET scan (November 4, 2007), and an MRI (November 12, 2007), the cancer medical team at Beth Israel Medical Center presented the following to me:

1. A second tumor was found on the MRI, not in my colon (which is why it wouldn't appear in the colonoscopy), but in the rectum, 3.5 centimeters (considered large).
2. The conclusion is that the particular cancer cells inside of me are highly resistant and certainly resistant to the state-of-the-art/industry mainline standard of chemotherapy, which is what I received (the FOLFOX regimen) from 2006 to March of 2007.
3. That I will undergo by the end of November *both* radiation (localized) and chemotherapy (throughout my entire body) to reduce size and spread *prior* to surgery (see more for projected schedule below).
4. That my condition is highly unique and problematic, to have *two* tumors, both of which seem unaffected by the best chemotherapy treatment.

Dr. Kozuch estimates that I have a 25 percent chance of living but hopes that with the combined radiation/chemo treatments, and surgery, and follow-up chemo/radiation postsurgery treatment to better my chances to 50 percent or higher.

He made it clear that more than likely, I will be unable to resume my professional life until the earliest mid-2008.

He also made it very clear that this is very experimental, murky, untested, uncharted area, with almost no precedents and verifiable data for course of treatment in my case. All to say that combining all five chemo drugs (for which FOLFOX was the best three out of the five) with something experimental and uncertifiable by the U.S. government (such as Avastin) may not be effective and may not be covered by *any* insurance and may cost around *half a million dollars*. He relayed how he has fought on behalf of other patients whom he wanted to get the total combined chemo mixture only to be turned down by CEOs of insurance companies.

He also conveyed possible side effects including allergic reaction, diarrhea, nausea, worsened peripheral neuropathy, and perhaps permanent nerve damage (and consequently major difficulty composing and playing the saxophone again).

The CT/PET scan taken on October 4 showed no visible sign of metastasis to vital organs (kidney, liver, lungs, heart, brain), a good sign; however, given the above, it is likely that metastasis has begun on the microscopic level, and more frequent scans (both CT/PET and MRI) will be required.

My medical care will now be centered at Beth Israel cancer treatment. A future memo will detail locations of my treatment and schedule.

The following doctors are part of this new medical team:

Surgeon: Dr. Antonio Picon

Chemo oncologist: Dr. Peter Kozuch

I haven't met with either but have scheduled for November 28, 2007 an appointment with a radiation oncologist: Dr. Kenneth Hu.

PROJECTED SCHEDULE

Immediately, I have postponed all of my activities from this point until mid–2008.

End of November, for six weeks, radiation (daily) and chemo therapy (every two weeks).

Mid-January 2008, for four to six weeks, allow body to recover.

Mid-February, surgery to remove both tumors; allow six weeks to heal.

Early April 2008, review with new CT/PET and MRI scans; ascertain further postsurgical treatment of additional radiation and/or chemotherapy.

Thank you to everyone who has called, e-mailed, written, and prayed for my beating the cancer's return. Mrs. Mary Sharp Cronson has again shown her generous and loving spirit and made a wonderful donation of $1,000. She continues to be my greatest supporter and patroness in the arts. I'd also thank other donations from Pam South (the CD player), Frances Goldin (for her $1,000 donation!), Su Zheng (for her generous $500 donation), the wonderful autographed book by Kip Fulbeck (*Part Hapa 100% Asian*), Weihua Zhang and Royal Hartigan for their gift of fruit, Dolly Veale, Bill Cole, Sarah Sully, and others. Your contributions are all very helpful.

Please stay in touch with Ann T. Greene to know when I will return home from the surgery. I will spend six to eight weeks recovering and would enjoy conversation, walks around my neighborhood, and just hanging out and maybe watching a DVD movie, listening to music, and enjoying a meal together.

But I feel *great*. I have used the six months since the end of chemo in March 2007 to rebuild myself, swimming, working out, bicycling, walking, and embarking upon a journey to eliminate *all* ego from within myself, getting off the treadmill of career aggrandizement, accumulation, and competition.

Excerpts of my *Diary of a Radical Cancer Warrior* have been published online in the latest KONCH, edited by Ishmael Reed: www.ishmaelreedpub.com.

We are embarking upon uncharted territory in the ongoing war against cancer. I will not know how I will be feeling, how much I can handle, etc. Please be understanding that if I cannot return people's phone calls, see you, or reply to your e-mails—we will figure out new strategy and tactics for this next rougher battle.

FIGHTING FRED HO TRIBUTE DECEMBER 16 BEFORE THE ONSLAUGHT BEGINS DECEMBER 17, 2007

"Bruce Lee defied tradition and earned the anger of narrow traditionalists who opposed his teaching of Chinese martial arts to non-Chinese, especially to Blacks. Fred Ho continues Lee's iconoclasm as the singular supporter of Blacks and Latinos in Asian martial arts today." (William Kevin "Doc" Savage, 2003)

On Sunday, December 16, 2007 at 2:00 PM, the American Museum of the Moving Image (located at Thirty-fifth Avenue at Thirty-sixth Street in Astoria, Queens; R or V train to Steinway Street or Q101 bus to Thirty-fifth Avenue) pays tribute to Fred Ho for his leading role in supporting and promoting blacks and Latinos in the Asian martial arts in the United States. The event is the world premiere of a new documentary film by Kamau Hunter and Jose Figueroa, *Urban Dragons* (2007, ninety minutes), examining the role and presence of blacks and Latinos in the martial arts in the United States. Following the screening will be a panel discussion with the filmmakers and the audience and the honoring of Fred Ho. In attendance will be some of the greatest living martial artists of today. The event is part of the *Sword and Fist* series curated by Warrington Hudlin. Please join us. For information, call 718-784-4520.

After a multitude of tests and doctors' meetings, a treatment plan has been developed. Because of the finding of the new second tumor and due to massive scar tissue from the surgery of the first colon cancer tumor in August of 2006, surgery has been postponed. Chemotherapy and radiation (drugs and information follows) will be administered in the hopes of reducing the tumors and containing cancer cell spread. Tests seem very hopeful and positive that cancer does not appear to have spread to my vital organs of kidneys, liver, lungs, heart, and brain.

The schedule for my combined chemotherapy and radiation treatment is as follows:

On Tuesday, December 11, I will receive my first chemo load-in of cetuximab (a.k.a. Erbitux), and additional x-rays to precisely confirm where radiation will be targeted.

On Monday, December 17, I will go to Beth Israel Hospital for 9:00 AM chemotherapy infusions while ingesting via tablets the chemo drug Xeloda daily Monday through Friday. Monday through Friday I will also have radiation.

I will have no treatments on weekends.

Close monitoring will be done of my side effects—which include nausea, diarrhea, hand-foot syndrome (extreme flaking, burning, chafing of the skin on my hands and my feet), possible loss of fertility, loss of hair, low blood counts, watery eyes and salivation, a possible metabolic, cholera-type of diarrhea called SN38, and possible mouth sores.

It is anticipated that after six weeks of this combined treatment that I will have/need six weeks off to recover. During this time I will be tested and evaluated and further treatment (surgery and/or more combined chemo/radiation) will be determined.

Besides two weeks of the flu, I have been feeling very good. I continue to exercise and swim regularly, go for daily walks of at least one mile, and I try to stay relaxed and rested. All my professional activities have all been postponed to fall 2008 or spring 2009, though I do want to complete a commission from Thomas Buckner for baritone voice and baritone saxophone, text to be written by Jayne Cortez, during my treatments.

I was very moved by the wonderful turnout of people who came to my last concert on October 25, celebrating the twenty-fifth anniversary of my band, the Afro Asian Music Ensemble. Robert Browning of the World Music Institute has been a wonderful friend and supporter. Thank you to the WMI and to everyone who came out and to the performers in both my band, the Afro Asian Music Ensemble, and the opening band, 3Z+. It was a joyful and terrific evening.

I continue to receive many letters, calls, and e-mails sending well wishes and love, as well as generous donations. Thank you to Idell Conaway, Cheryl Higashida, Nick and Laura Unger, Dolly Veale, Sylvie Degiez/Wayne Lopes, Rebecca Lazier, and Miyoshi Smith for their cash gifts in this recent period. Tom Buckner and Kamala Cesar gave a very generous donation of $1,000.

Below is the medical analysis and treatment plan.

HO, Fred DOB: 08/10/57 IDX MRN: 2337332
Emergency contact: Dr. Florence Houn
November 14, 2007 INITIAL BETH ISRAEL MEDICAL
ONCOLOGY CONSULTATION NOTE

DISEASE: Pelvic recurrence of adenocarcinoma of the sigmoid colon.

HISTORY OF THE PRESENT ILLNESS: The patient is a fifty-year-old gentleman found to have a sporadic case of adenocarcinoma of the colon, rectosigmoid, and underwent surgery August 29, 2006. Presenting symptomatology was lower GI bleeding and diarrhea. He underwent an R0 resection of a pathologic T4 B N1 (1/22 lymph nodes replaced by metastatic carcinoma with extension into surrounding mesenteric adipose tissue. The proximal and distal margins are negative for tumor, but no specific comment on circumferential margin status. He completed twelve cycles of adjuvant modified FOLFOX March 2007 under the care of Dr. Dilip Patel (718) 470-4454. Treatment was complicated by grade two to three neuropathy from January until June 2007. He also had what sounds like an allergic reaction possibly to the oxaliplatinum, which was successfully managed by swelling oxaliplatinum infusion rate. He has persistent grade 1 neuropathy, but this does not interfere with his musicianship; he is a professional saxophonist.

Unfortunately by July 2007 he developed recurrent diarrhea and bright red blood per rectum. Colonoscopy September 24, 2007, showed a friable lesion 15 cm from the anal verge. Correlative biopsy, however, showed nonspecific colitis, no evidence of cancer. He was evaluated by Dr. Antonio Picon (surgical oncologist Beth Israel Medical Center) October 17, 2007. MRI referral to Dr. David Robbins for EUS, endoscopy, and repeat biopsy recommended. The patient's situation was presented to the GI Tumor Board Beth Israel Medical Center November 12, 2007. Attendance included

Dr. Warren Enker colorectal surgery, Dr. Antonio Picon surgical oncology, Dr. Joseph Martz colorectal surgery, Dr. Kenneth Hu radiation oncology. Consensus was that because the MRI showed the sigmoid neoplasm within the pelvis as well as a presacral mass suspicious for regional nodal metastasis versus mesenteric implant. Consensus was to proceed with neoadjuvant chemoradiation therapy prior to definitive resection.

SOCIAL HISTORY: He is a professional saxophonist. He is a lifelong nonsmoker, nondrinker, nondrug user.

REVIEW OF SYSTEMS: Positive symptoms limited to frequent bowel movement and bright red blood per rectum. He has no symptomatology to suggest anemia and no weight loss. Additional eight systems reviewed and are unremarkable.

PHYSICAL EXAMINATION: Well-appearing gentleman and no acute distress. Height: Not documented, weight: 218 lbs; BP: 120/80' pulse: 78; pain: 0; temp: 97. HEENT- PERRL, EOMI, OP: Normal; Lungs: Bilaterally CTA/P; Heart: Regular rhythm, no gallops, or rubs. Abdomen: Soft, nontender, nondistended, no masses, organomegaly, or ascites. Extremities: No clubbing, cyanosis, or edema. Lymphatic survey: There is no cervical, supraclavicular, axillary, epitrochlear, or inguinal adenopathy. Neurological exam: Normal mental acuity. Cranial nerves II–XII, motor and cerebellar function intact.

PATHOLOGY DATA: Surgical pathology report North Shore University Hospital at Forest Hills rectosigmoid colon— adenocarcinoma of the colon, moderately differentiated pT4 N1 (1/22 lymph nodes positive for metastatic carcinoma, which extends into the surrounding mesenteric adipose tissue. Proximal and distal margins negative for tumor circumferential margin status not mentioned, lymphovascular invasion not mentioned.

IMAGING DATA:
October 05, 2007, CT/PET scan skull through thighs.

October 05, 2007 North Shore Long Island Jewish Health Care System: Findings highly suspicious for recurrent colon cancer at the sigmoid anastomotic site. Small focus of mild hypermetabolism in the rectum maximum SUV of 6.4 without corresponding abnormality on CT scan.

Beth Israel Medical Center November 11, 2007, pelvic MRI with contrast: Findings most consistent with sigmoid neoplasm with mild multifocal extension due to the pericolonic fat.

Focal left presacral mass very suspicious for spread of disease. Mass immediately abuts the piriformis muscle.

Plaquelike soft tissue thickening of the sigmoid mesentery either desmoplastic reaction or spread of disease.

Mildly enlarged heterogenous prostate. Notably presacral mass measures $3.5 \times 2.2 \times 1.7$ cm. This probably involves the mesorectal fashion near its junction within the peritoneal reflection as well as the presacral space.

Outside colonoscopy report to cecum: Recurrent friable lesion at 15 cm. Remainder of colon is reportedly unremarkable. Colonoscopist, Richard Emanuel, MD, Forest Hills Medical, 96-10 Metropolitan Avenue, Forest Hills, NY 11375.

LABORATORY DATA:
October 31, 07, CBC/CMP: CMP-unremarkable, normal liver function profile, albumen 4.4, WBC 5.0, hemoglobin 15.6, MCV 92.8, platelets 284, CEA 0.8, PT/PTT—unremarkable.

IMPRESSION/PLAN: Sixty-minute consultation with the patient. The next day a thirty-minute conversation with the patient's sister, Florence Houn, MD, who is a preventive oncologist in Bethesda, Maryland. The patient and his sister understand and agree with the following:

Pelvic recurrence of colon cancer with possible presacral nodal metastasis. They understand that confirmatory biopsy is required before any neoadjuvant intent chemoradiation can begin. Assuming pelvic recurrence of colon adenocarcinoma is confirmed, the November 12, 2007, GI Tumor Board consensus was to proceed with neoadjuvant chemoradiation therapy prior to resection. Given the fact that his colon cancer recurred during FOLFOX, he should be thought of as having colon cancer primarily refractory to this regimen. Therefore, non-cross resistant chemotherapy needs to be partnered with radiation therapy in order to optimize not just local control, but also address possible distant micrometastases. Standard treatment for patients with colorectal cancer that is resistant to FOLFOX is irinotecan with cetuximab. In order to optimize radiation sensitivity, I would add Xeloda to this combination. Evidence supporting the feasibility of preoperative chemoradiation therapy with irinotecan, capecitabine, and cetuximab comes from Hong et al. *Journal of Clinical Oncology* 2007 ASCO annual meeting proceedings part 1 volume 25 #18S, abstract #4045. The regimen consisted of cetuximab 400 mg/M2 on day 6 one week prior to radiation therapy followed by weekly cetuximab 250 mg/M2, irinotecan 40 mg/M2 and capecitabine 1650 mg/M2 BID weekdays only during radiation. The potential side effects of this regimen including, but not limited to nausea, vomiting, acne like rash over face, back and chest, which can be severe, dry skin, perionychial cracking along the fingernail edges, cutaneous toxicity along the perineum, low blood counts including the potential need for growth factor transfusion support, fevers, allergic reactions, hand-foot syndrome, mouth sores, and diarrhea reviewed. He is familiar with these drugs and was given literature on each of them.

Predisposition to iron deficiency anemia—he is encouraged to start taking one iron tablet with one vitamin C tablet daily. He understands to stop this medication the first sign of significant constipation.

Confirmatory biopsy with Dr. David Robbins.

ASAP consult with Kenneth Hu radiation oncology.

Follow up in this office in two weeks so that plans for chemoradiation therapy can be finalized. In the meantime we will obtain preauthorization for all of the above-mentioned systemic therapies.

Peter Kozuch, MD

cc: Kenneth Hu, MD, via e-mail

cc: Antonio Picon, MD, via e-mail

cc: David Robbins, MD, via e-mail

cc: Dilip Patel, MD, Long Island Jewish Oncology Service 27-05 Seventy-sixth Avenue

DIARY 13: THE ULTIMATE URBAN DRAGON FIGHTS THE GAUNTLET OF HADES

December 19, 2007

The screening of *Urban Dragons* (a ninety-minute documentary film by Kamau Hunter and Jose Figueroa) at the Museum of the Moving Image, curated by Warrington Hudlin, was glorious. It was an honor to be in the presence of the so many African American and Latino American living legend martial artists. I was presented with a wonderful plague that reads as follows:

> In acknowledgement of the Masters presented in this film *Urban Dragons: Black and Latino Masters of Chinese Martial Arts* the producers proudly present this award of excellence to Fred Ho, martial arts pioneer, in honor of the genius in your revelations of the true international face of martial arts today with African and Latino personalities all benefiting from and upholding the best traditions of Chinese martial arts in urban America.
>
> Your revolutionary and creative focus on meshing Chinese martial arts with jazz in theater is without peer and of a vision that speaks to the unity of men bound by an ancient warrior's code personified by the individuals profiled in *Urban Dragons*.
>
> Your overwhelming dedication to righting injustices with the heart of a warrior, the intellect of a philosopher, and the righteousness of the spiritual, makes you, to all those that celebrate what you stand for, Fred Ho—the Ultimate Urban Dragon.

THE DESCENT INTO HELL HAS BEGUN

The combination of chemotherapy and radiation treatments has begun. The path to hell is like a gauntlet, unpredictable and volatile, and most certainly brutal. The doors to the chambers of hell include some familiar and some unfamiliar demons:

Nausea: been there in the first war and presently equipped to fight it with medications and rest.

Diarrhea: been there in the first war and presently equipped to fight it with medications, rest, and my sister Flora's special congee.

Loopiness and fatigue: rest and sleep and deep breathing.

Watery eyes: let it pour.

Slow hair growth or complete hair loss: eliminate vanity.

Hand-Foot Syndrome (extreme blistering, cracking of the skin on hands, arms, feet and legs): special creams and feet and hand wear, minimal dish washing by hand, special attention to bathing.

Rashes, acne: eliminate vanity, do not use dehydrating acne or rash medication, be patient and wait for these side effects to pass.

Depression: immerse in love.

Dehydration: drink a variety of liquids including high-quality mineral water, teas, juices without pulp. Wake up constantly to keep hydrated. Constantly hydrate my skin with good lotions. Use a humidifier in my apartment.

How to Wage the War to Win

1. Recognize that the internal war inside my body at the cellular level is going to be far more severe, the analogy is like the first war was conventional warfare with standard weapons as well as with weapons of mass destruction (chemo); this new war will be all of what was used before, though different weapons

of mass destruction combined with chemical and radioactive weaponry including star wars systems. Every Monday for the next six weeks will be the major offensive, an all-day unremitting onslaught, starting at 9:00 AM radiation zapping and 11:00 AM chemo bombardment (alternating between Erbitux only, a three-hour treatment, to Erbitux and Irinotecan, four to four and a half hours combined treatment). The goal: reduce and/or wipe out tumors and kill as many spreading, circulating microscopic cancer cells throughout my body. Thursdays to Fridays will be radiation with orally ingested chemo medication.

2. Apply all methods and principles developed and learned from first war including the following:
   a. Continue on the journey to eliminate ego (to accept even the smallest kernel of truth no matter how it is delivered or who is the messenger).
   b. Stay off the treadmill of career, acquisitiveness, comparison and competition.
   c. Nutrition, hydration, oxygenation, and *love* are my personal special weapons.
3. To give and to receive *love*. The best armor in the gauntlet through Hades is finding joy and fun. The many friends who have joined me in the hospital, taken me home, fed me, shared jokes, laughter, stories, walks, etc., have filled the brief moments I have of physical normalcy with radiance and strength. *A special listserv report will be sent soon by Magdalena Gómez on our recent fun escapades together, including some fun photos.*

How to Help

Many people inquire about how to help beyond donating money. I have made a list below:

Donating beverages. High-grade mineral water (flat or with carbonation) such as Trader Joe's Blu Italy, San Faustino, Pellegrino. Avoid: Perrier. Also, rice milk (Trader Joe's is best and lowest price), mango nectar, ingredients to make smoothies; teas (noncaffeine, no sweeteners).

Donating cooked food. Miso soup with tofu and seaweed and scallions, cabbage; applesauce (no sugars/sweeteners); pancake mix and real maple syrup; pasta salads; potato leek soup; congee; bananas; cooked beet dishes; pork loin, pork chops; lamb chops; pizza; tofu dishes with cooked veggies; avocado; glazed carrots; dinner rolls, and refined wheats.

Other ways to help. Driving, especially on Mondays (see below), from treatments to social events, movies and arts events, botanical gardens.

Companionship for Monday Treatments. Taking notes, interfacing with hospital staff and physicians, running errands for bottled water, snacks/lunch; talking with me when I'm awake.

Home visits. I can only see people Thursdays and Fridays after 1:00 PM and weekends by e-mail appointments. These visits can include conversation, helping with errands, light housecleaning, etc. Please be aware that my condition may worsen considerably and alterations to appointments might be done last minute. Please also note that my appearance may deteriorate as well.

Intimate assistance. Body lotion application; massages; hydration application (via special creams and ointments I provide) to hands, feet, buttocks (for radiation burns), stomach. If you have a problem with my nudity, please do not offer.

There are many loving thank-yous:

To Robert Amory, a great portrait photographer (www.lightofothers.com) who took a beautiful head shot of me and who donated $500 to my war against cancer;

To my father, Franklin Wu Houn, for his contribution of $1,000;

Also thanks to Diane Fujino, Bill Mullen and Robin D.G. Kelley for their contributions toward my collection of selected writings, *Wicked Theory, Naked Practice*: *Selected Writings on Radical Political and Cultural Theory* by Fred Ho, which will be published by the University of Minnesota Press (thanks to Adam Bruenner, my editor there).

DIARY 14: TRANSCENDENCE AND
TRANSFORMATION IS WHAT WE MUST EXPECT

December 25, 2007

My dear friends,

It is not how hard you hit, it is how hard you get hit and keep moving forward.

I've completed two weeks (out of six, four more to go) of combined chemo and radiation treatments. The side effects I have are diarrhea, terrible zits and rash (I'm starting to look like a leper), and extreme fatigue. Some days I sleep for sixteen hours. My ability to even do e-mails or return people's phone calls has fallen. Please excuse this lapse.

Here are some interesting occurrences for the past two weeks:

Wednesday, December 26, 2007: For my radiation treatment today, I tried visualization while getting zapped on the cold steel board. I visualized myself stomach-down resting on a surfboard with gently undulating waves rocking me. It was fantastic! I was able to "transport" myself to the ocean and the soft lapping waves helped me to rest and relax in the perfectly still, confined position I have to be in for ten minutes for the treatment. I must admit that I had skepticism about visualization, but now that I've attained it, I am a supporter.

I received a letter from Susan Dadian, programming director of Chamber-Music America, conferring my band, the Afro Asian Music Ensemble, as an awardee of the CMA/ASCAP Awards for Adventurous Programming of Contemporary Music, to be present at their annual convention on Saturday, January 5, 2008, at the

Westin Times Square Hotel in the Gershwin Ballroom from 1:30 PM to 3:30 PM. I will be afforded an opportunity to speak from a panel of other awardees.

My Afro Asian Music Ensemble celebrated its twenty-fifth anniversary this past October 2007. For the twenty-five years, there are special people who have been consistent supporters of the band that I would like to recognize and thanks, including Robert and Helene Browning of the World Music Institute, all the friends at the Brooklyn Academy of Music (from Joe Melillo, Karen Brooks-Hopkins, Pat Scully, Alice Bernstein, of course Harvey Lichtenstein!), Limor Tomer, Giovanni Bonandrini and Soul Note Records in Italy, Mary Sharp Cronson, Laura Greer and the Apollo Theater, John Killacky, Chuck Helm, Philip Bither, Julie Voight, and the fifteen-plus years of association with the Walker Art Center, John Duffy and all the friends that have journeyed with us from Meet the Composer, Joseph Franklin, Marty and Helene Khan, Joseph Yoon.

The point of technique is to have no technique.

In my war against cancer, it became crystal clear to me why I have been put on planet Earth: to create performance works that no one will or can create and to compose music for musicians no one will or can write music for.

I'd like to sing the praises of two very special people whose cooking expresses the deliciousness of their souls: Brooke Stephens and Margaret Porter Troupe (which makes her husband, Quincy, one of the luckiest men alive!). Brooke's turkey, gravy, stuffing, soup, mac-and-cheese have been the best I've ever tasted. And I'm a constant fan of Margaret's exciting Harlem Arts Salon series presented from her home featuring great writers, artists, and intellects and her savory buffets. Fantastico!

Boards don't hit back.

TWO WEEKS DONE, FOUR MORE TO GO!

Week 1. My first combined radiation and chemo all-day treatment at Beth Israel Medical Center was companioned by Magdalena Gomez, taking copious medical notes, interfacing with all staff and making me comfortable, fetching me water and food, and being such a terrific pal. By week's end, I was completely hammered. Zits breaking out on my face and head, sleeping constantly, exhausted, absolutely zero mental and physical energy not even enough to read two sentences or even watch TV for two minutes. Zonked and beaten down. Some diarrhea began on Sunday. The treatments are every weekdays with Saturdays and Sundays off.

If you don't hit it, it won't fall.

Week 2. From this point every Monday is an all-day in-hospital treatment. The second week all-day treatment was covered ably by Parker Pracjek, who brought her own goodies including bottled water, cooked veggie burgers, fruits. She also took me home in a cab after the treatments.

Don't take things personally, take things seriously.

Many people have sent a bounty of information on alternative and complementary cancer treatments. I have had a much harder time now that the side effects have been hammering me to spend much time reviewing all the web links and materials, but I eventually do get a chance to peruse and evaluate the leads. The information and treatment offering I have become most favorable toward was sent to me by Dr. Greta Shames-Dawson for Dr. Charles Simone (www.drsimone.com). Dr. Simone's familiarity with the data of a broad range of tests and studies, his due diligence on alternative, and complementary methods make for very solid treatment evaluations. He also doesn't seem to be self-promoting in a monetarily driven way. While I have a far more radical critique of the American health care system and the cancer industry (big pharma, multilevel marketing schemes, etc., discussed critically in my cancer war diary during the war's first stage from fall

2006 to March 2007) than Dr. Simone, I believe his due diligence on existing medical science as well as the alternative/complementary field is very thorough.

Conflict can't be killed; it can only be resolved.

The outpouring of love and support from everyone continues to fortify me during days when I can barely open my eyelids and pull myself out of bed.

Special thanks to longtime dear friends from Kaneohe, Hawaii, Richard Hamasaki and Jennifer Dang for their financial and cultural gifts.

To David Kastin for his financial gift and for writing a cultural studies analysis of my *Voice of the Dragon* work.

To Woody, Annetta, and Miles Igou for the batch of Floridian oranges.

Thanks to Brooke Stephens for her donation of a humidifier and for being the chef of a delicious Xmas dinner and hostess of the mostest!

To Dr. Royal Hartigan, longtime friend and musical colleague, one of the world's great drummers, for his generous financial gift.

Compromise is unacceptable; transcendence and transformation is what we must expect and accept.

DIARY 15: HOPE FOR THE BEST, PREPARE FOR THE WORST, UNDERSTANDING THE INTEGRATED STRATEGY AND TACTICS OF A PROTRACTED CANCER WAR

January 8, 2008

Dear beloved friends,

Three weeks done, starting the fourth week with three more weeks to go in the combined chemo/radiation treatment.

The first stage in my cancer war with solely the FOLFOX chemo protocol began October 5, 2006, and ended March 10, 2007. In that war, I had three straight days of chemo and eleven days off for six months. During that time, I was fortunate to have anywhere from one to eight, maybe even nine, days of sufficient energy to practice my saxophone, compose music, write, exercise, organize and produce, socialize more (such as an almost-weekly Fatback Fan Club outing in which some friends ventured forth into Queens to check out new culinary gems and other gatherings).

However, this round, which is for six weeks, I have been smashed and hammered by a much more severe protocol that includes all Mondays combined radiation and three chemo drugs and then Tuesdays and Fridays combined radiation and one chemo drug. My Saturdays and Sundays are off, but I have yet to have sufficient energy to stay awake for more than seven hours continuously.

I have tried to not take powerful prescription medications to fight nausea, diarrhea, fatigue, and have preferred natural alternatives such as my sister's congee recipe for diarrhea, sleep and rest, hydration. Many of these medications are steroids and while I may get a "push" of energy and am able to stay awake and do some things, in the end, I collapse from exhaustion from this boosted push.

Some of you have read my current diary entries and have shared with me your views ranging from being highly critical of what you view as my usage of conventional treatments (chemo and radiation) and not enough reliance upon alternatives. Some have been gentler and offer ample materials on alternative and complementary proposals. I appreciate all the efforts because I know you are all my beloved friends, wish me wellness and everything beneficial, and have the ultimate respect of allowing me to make decisions about my life and will not allow your egos or your philosophical precepts to make our differences or disagreements into conflicts. I know you love and respect me, and I know you know I love and respect all of you.

I want to particularly acknowledge the abundant articles and information sent to me by Dr. Greta Shames-Dawson, Daystarr Chou, Beverly Naidus and her husband Bob, Peter Rachleff, Bob Lederer, and others who share with me their personal struggles with cancer themselves or the struggles they know very personally, such as Stephanie Hughley.

Because of the unrelenting hammering of this current treatment, I have not been able to elaborate as much of a combined philosophical and practical explanation of my strategic plan in this current stage of the cancer war, simply because I have little energy even to sit for a few minutes and type something like what I'm typing now (tonight, as I type this, I did take the steroid-based medications).

PRINCIPLES AND FINDING PARTICLES OF TRUTH

I want to request from my blog administrators, Ann T. Greene and Magdalena Gómez, to allow all on our Warriors for Fred LISTSERV to be able to send comments to everyone on the LISTSERV should you feel you want to comment on what I will say below. Again, my principle is accept any particles of truth no matter who the messenger or how the message is delivered. I want to offer unconditional thanks to all who feel they can and want to contribute to my education, to correct me, to differ and present substitution prescriptions or protocols. Your comments can and should range from the philosophical to the immediately practical and strategically effective (i.e., a prescription or path for victory).

First, my strategy may be called "integrative," which differs from conventional/allopathic and alternative and complementary.

Conventional/allopathic relies upon the Western medical establishment's protocols and precepts (data, testing, methodology, etc.). I don't do this.

Alternative relies upon nonconventional/nonallopathic (i.e., Western) medical science, mostly on supplements, nutrition, herbs, acupuncture, and other medicinal products (noni juice, mangosteen, Essiac, etc.) and practices (*chi-gong*, visualization, reiki, meditation, etc.). I don't do this.

Complementary relies upon the Western medical science but supplements it with the alternative methods and products. I don't do this.

Now the Western medical science has something they describe as "integrative," which in their meaning is interdisciplinary within the realms of their canon: combining gastroenterology with colorectal surgery with chemo-oncology with radiation oncology with nutrition with psycho-physical with the spiritual/faith, etc. The weakness in this conception, while a more preferred organizing principle than the fragmentation of disciplines (which is more of what could be described as what I had in the first round of the war from 2006 to mid-2007), nonetheless, is predominantly within the Western medical science canon, though certain physicians and practitioners are more broadly accepting of other practices and products, some giving credibility to practitioners who have little or no training at all within the allopathic canon.

Here is what I mean by *integrative*: try everything as long as there is a provable argument (subject to any verification and collaboration of details) and isn't transparently profiteering (e.g., multilevel marketing schemes, super drugs that cost $250,000 that don't cure but only in their own clinical trials simply on the average prolong life for a little over six months on the average but with mostly a horrible quality of life with awful side effects) and finally, not propagandizing that cancer *in general* can be cured (the magic bullet) because I have rejected that premise as explained in the diaries 1 to 15 (simply, the causes are myriad and part of the very fabric of modern industrial capitalist existence, and therefore no single cure will ever be found, but a multiplicity of cures can be implemented necessary to the replacement of modern industrial capitalist existence with another mode of existence). I accept some propaganda that certain people and their cancers can be cured, but that a definitive remission rate of over 85 percent for all cancers at all stages, which I would liberally grant to be a cure, isn't possible given the systemic causes. I grant that for certain types of cancers at certain lower stages that conventional protocols have statistical verification to grant general efficacy.

That was how I got the original FOLFOX treatment for stage 3b colorectal cancer. In the clinical trials a few years ago, the FDA was compelled by ethical mandate to approve this protocol as the mainline treatment for my type and stage of cancer because so many of the thousands of trial participants were showing marked improvements, including remission, that the trials ended early and the protocol was conferred as the new industry standard. Certainly in my case, it was ineffective. And to make matters worse, a new tumor was found, undetected in the first round, quite probably because an MRI scan wasn't done (CT/PET scans were done).

Conventional approaches have very little data, trial evidence, and other indicators for recurrence of cancer across the board. While no one on the allopathic side has stated my condition to be metastatic (meaning beyond localized), I go by the old-school warrior principle: "Hope for the best; prepare for the worst."

It is difficult to say whether the chemo in the first round added more harm, as it certainly didn't do any good (was ineffective, even admitted by the allopathic doctors).

Here is a brutal irony I am struggling with: perhaps the complementary and alternative approaches I took (the "fighting on the cellular level" protocol I offered in round one of nutrition, hydration, oxygenation, and *love*) may have had a duality of both helping and harming. The former by warding off the worst side effects and being very effective in maintaining my strength, spirit, and some aspects of my immune system, but *also* somehow "feeding" the cancer cells. I am still very unclear on all this, as it is a profoundly disturbing concept. But I remain ready to reevaluate *everything*.

Let me explain. There are a lot of "perhaps-es" in this still-formulating thinking on my part:

Perhaps the many and varied fruit juices I drank, provided strong and good antioxidants but at the same time, their natural sugars fed the cancer cells;

Perhaps all methods of oxygenation of cells, including immersion in oxygen chambers (something Michael Jackson was ridiculed/lampooned for doing), can not be done and is untestable and impossible given the state of all medical sciences (allopathic and nonallopathic). In my case, I did *chi-gong* deep breathing, reiki, surround myself with plants, and regular visits to the rainforest chamber of the Brooklyn Botanical Garden). I didn't do the oxygen chamber.

Perhaps stopping to eat red meat, reducing animal fats, preferring a more raw food, Mediterranean and East Asian (MSG-free) diet, while nutritiously powerful, still could have continued to "feed" the cancer cells (meaning I have not changed enough of my diet/nutritional plan).

The one component of my last strategy I will not concede as possibly "feeding" the cancer cells is *love*, which filled me with joy and happiness, never letting me feel I was "sick" or despondent or sad or overwhelmed. I cannot surrender to fatalism and leave my fate to statistics, solely to prayer and even to an all-powerful being. *Love* is what fuels my fight to win. And really, life is not worth living if there isn't *love*. Some have misconstrued my conceptualizing the struggle against cancer as a "war" or "fighting" trying to persuade me to conceive of the struggle as one of "nurturing" my body and spirit, of "breathing" and letting go of the unnecessary and unwanted, etc. I don't counterpose these two conceptions. Indeed I believe they are two sides of the same coin. Or as Che Guevara said, "At the risk of sounding ridiculous, I believe a revolution is guided by a great feeling of love" (he was referring to love of the people, not just to specific persons, or family, or community, or friends—but to a profound love that believes in the liberation of the people as a revolutionary transformative power as necessary, prerequisite and unconditional in the struggle to cure cancer by ridding the world of capitalism and its toxic waste, overconsumption, ecological degradation and exploitative physical, social, cultural, and psychic processes).

So, *integration* in my conception, is the strategy and usage/experimentation with everything, relying upon one conception for a time though always combining with a range of other concepts/methodologies, shifting to another, reconfiguring emphases, a totally aggressive application of experimentation, innovation, determination, and principled directional shifts (principles as elaborated above as provable arguments, rejection of blatant exploitative profiteering schemes, magic bullet-hyped cure). This includes possible shifts such as going abroad and using integrative strategies of other countries' medical and treatment sciences; exiting modern industrial society altogether and deciding to live the rest of my life in as near-pristine rain forest conditions as possible for the current stage of our planet; etc. I am investigating all options. You can offer ones I haven't thought of, and please make a provable argument as best as you can.

THE DUE DILIGENCE OF A PROVABLE ARGUMENT: GIVE ME THE DETAILS

Let me elaborate on what I consider to be a *provable argument*. I don't necessarily mean clinical trial data, studies, etc. My conditions for provable argument won't rely solely upon personal or hearsay anecdotes ("this worked for me or someone I know well") *unless* since I vow to welcome all truths, no matter how microscopic, as long as I can ascertain or investigate some degree of the details (who, what, where, when, how, duration, actual practices, or products, etc.). This is not to dissuade anyone from contributing anecdotal information so long as they really try to get the fullest details. I hope all of you regard our friendship as worthy of that effort. Those are my simple grounds for a provable argument: do the best due diligence for me as you can so I can best continue that due diligence. *And* balance those anecdotes (especially the more phenomenal or seemingly-miraculous ones) with the opposite: cases where that practice or product has *failed* (with as much detail of course). The alternative product and treatment propaganda abounds with these heart-warming success stories. Transparently, I have never read a balanced account that cites caveats, failures, disappointment testimonials. At least the allopathic literature stipulates qualifications, exceptions, narrowness of range of claims, and failures and death rates. The truth is that there can be no cure to cancer as long as capitalism exists, that is a Fred Ho challenge and contradiction and qualification to the Ralph Mosses, the Dr. Charles Simones, the Gary Nulls, etc. (My apologies if my claim, challenge, conflict, contradiction, qualification sounds egotistical, but that is my particle or morsel/molecule of truth, and I hope all will accept my particle or morsel/molecule as I would yours!)

As a contribution to all of you who are Warriors for Fred (which I term and describe interchangeably also as my "circle of love"), I would like to ask you to check out the following from two fellow warriors/ love circlists, who are also very special friends to me:

Bill Fletcher's new book (with Fernando Gaspin), *Solidarity Divided: The Crisis in Organized Labor and a New Path for Social Justice*).

Magdalena Gómez's benefit reading/performance for Doctors for Global Health (www.dghonline.org) on Friday, November 25, 2008, from 8:00 PM to 11:00 PM at the Bruckner Bar and Grill (www.brucknerbar.com) in El Bronx.

I'd like to offer *kudos* to the Free Mumia forces for very soundly countering the pro-death to Mumia forces in their latest mainstream media offensive.

I'd like to offer *right ons* to the expanding support for people's attorneys Michael and Evelyn Warren in their battle for justice for the police brutality they were subjected to.

The above two causes are especially dear to me, as are the comrades.

And as always, I'd like to give thanks to the following people for their very generous financial gifts:

Q Moct and Jose Figueroa, Frances Goldin, Peter Rachleff and Beth Cleary, Leon Yankwich, and Elaine Fong.

And to the many people who have sent cards and well wishes: Idell Conaway, Baraka Sele, Dolly Veale (for the DVD and tea as well), Ken Chu, Ricardo Gomes and Maria, Eric Mann for the "organic intellectual" care package, Kay and Jack Shelemay for the fresh fruits, Shoba Narayana for the CDs, Sean Lewis for cooking a bountiful and delicious lunch, Jennifer Kidwell for the whole-grain bread and joyful company, and so many others.

Finally, thanks to Gladys Serrano for joining me at Beth Israel Medical Center for the Monday, January 7, 2008, combined all-day treatment, and to Judith Sloan for driving me home afterward.

And if I failed to acknowledge anyone, my profoundest apologies: my lapse is due to the constant state of being smashed and my inability at most times to even have enough energy to make a note to myself to cite your help.

DIARY 16: THE ROAD THROUGH HELL IS LOVE

January 30, 2008

This is my final week in hell before my six- to eight-week recovery period in which, I hope, most of the side effects will have subsided and gone away, and I can return to some normality, prepare myself for surgery to cut out the two tumors (colon-rectal and pelvic). After which, it is projected, that I will need another six weeks to recover from surgery and most likely proceed with another combined round of chemo-radiation. It looks like a good part of the first half of 2008 will be engaged in this war as my primary focus.

My personal gauntlet through hell has been extreme daily fatigue, three or four days of agonizing diarrhea, eruption of zits all over my face, head, neck and chest and lower buttocks, and this past week, skin breakage on one of my left hand fingers that resulted in infection (for which I am on antibiotic medication).

During this period, I have learned of other people I know who have been diagnosed with cancer. The details in my diaries are to hopefully serve as useful anticipation of what to expect, preparation for how to fight, and inspiration and understanding for a warrior spirit.

I live alone, so my time in hell was only very partially experienced/ observed by others. Most of the time, I was facing it on my own. However, my dear friend Peggy Choy did come and visit and spent a lot of time with me in the middle of this onslaught. She stayed for one night sleeping on the coach in my living room, and I am sorry her sleep was constantly interrupted by the agony of my hours of diarrhea and middle-of-the night darts to the toilet. It would have been tough for anyone to endure hearing the sounds of my stomach pains, the explosive blasts of my bowel movements throughout the whole night until 5:00 AM when I seem to have expunged everything and slept finally from exhaustion.

Peggy also did a lot of chores I had no energy to do, from helping with cooking, cleaning my entire apartment including bathroom and kitchen, doing laundry, helping do my end of year taxes, running errands, wash dishes, taking out garbage, and recycling. This is a something very few people have witnessed: my complete incapacity to do even basic chores.

And she graciously accepted how awful company I am during this hell. Barely able to speak audibly, to have the mental energy to even explain things, to simply be catatonic, or asleep almost all of the time. We both got hooked on the new TV show *Terminator: The Sarah Connor Chronicles* because we like women warrior characters. She asked to watch on DVD the movie *Terminator 2*. I put it on, but had to go to my bedroom after a few minutes since I couldn't muster the energy to stay awake and view it with her. Most of the time all I could do was get up, answer the door to let her in to my apartment, give her a list of things I needed to have her do for me, sleep, and wake up when she was ready to leave to see her out (after the first night, she stayed with her sister across the hall in my building).

WHAT IS TRUST?

I have learned something on this concept, especially the distinction/ differentiation between control versus trust. I used to rely on control, my capability to get a lot done and at a high standard, to demand that from all with whom I'm engaged. I would get upset with or disappointed in people who flaked out or couldn't deliver or come through with promises or commitments. I was iron clad about holding that standard to myself. What I've come to understand is that trust operates precisely when control is absent or entirely in question/ impossible to attain. One must trust people to deliver or come through when one is completely unable to control any of the choices or circumstances.

I was a control freak, as some might describe me, especially during the carcinogenic period of my life and I believe the cancer took hold of me internally through a combination of conditions: the internal combination of a life and attitude locked onto the treadmill and the diet that went along with this path. Control was part of what I wrongly perceived I needed to have to acquire and accumulate, though comparatively speaking to most Americans, I was pretty anti consumerist, anti acquisitive, anti obsessive about a lot of things and selfish satisfaction indices. But nonetheless, I equated more with better. I didn't realize that world inequality won't end until most of the first world can learn to live closer to that of most people in the third world. That the concept of technological and consumerist horn-of-plenty utopia is toxic and unsustainable.

As one struggles for mastery/discipline over one's path and circumstances, there is a sifting, culling, vetting process, mostly taught from learning from mistakes (both from others and from ones I commit). There are two paths to this process of mastery: on the one hand, implementing greater management (more precise agreements, higher proficiency requirements, longer lists of dos and don'ts, etc.). On the other, transcending the former into a circle of trust that becomes one's entire community. I am much happier and fulfilled by the latter. But the latter is a process attained by the struggle of the former.

For example, my professional artistic collaborators are all my close personal friends. To say we are a team only partially captures the spirit and trust we all have. But that came to happen after years of struggle, sometimes difficult and tense. Now I feel no need to have contracts, etc. And they bring to the artistic collaboration exciting challenges to my work and my concepts that makes all of us better. The role of competitive egos is completely absent. The respect and trust we share spreads to newer collaborators and performers, creating a community of standards, respect and trust that makes all better and hence our working together a joy and constant learning-transforming experience.

I hope I have communicated the general idea of what I have learned. I'm still learning, so I welcome comments and feedback.

CONSTANT LOVE AND THANKS TO EVERYONE'S GENEROUS SPIRIT

Big thanks to the very generous donations from Jesse Wardlow (an ol' college buddy); Pamela South (with a beautiful photo of herself and her daughter Ava); Quincy and Margaret Troupe for visiting and bringing wonderful food; Debreh Gilbert and Bob Hawks for companioning me on Monday, January 14, and for driving me home;

the generous financial gift along with some music from Woody Igou and his family; to Claude Marks (www.freedomarchives.org) for the wonderful CD *Words Like Freedom: Paul Robeson*; financial gifts from Miyoshi Smith (again!); and from folks at the Labor/Community Strategy Center (www.thestrategycenter.org) Eric Mann, Kelly and Patricia Archbold, Francisca Porchas, Sunyoung Yang, and Tammy Luu; the huge care packages sent by Limor Tomer.

And to the small contingent that came to my place on Saturday, January 12, including Peggy Choy visiting from Wisconsin, Ann Greene, and Mark O'Ferrall, Lois Greene and the wisest twenty-one-month-old person, baby Lilli—they all helped clean house, repair my kitchen cabinets, lotion me from head to feet, cooked, ran errands, and showed me the beauty and joy of friendship. I am constantly impressed and amazed at baby Lilli, who as the Greene family was preparing to leave my place, not only fetched her own shoes (which she isn't able yet to put on), but the shoes of all the adults in her family and making the effort to help them on with their shoes. The word "precocious" and "precious" can only simultaneously describe her.

Many thanks to Femi Agana for companioning me to my final in-hospital treatments on Monday, January 22, and to Mark O'Ferrall for driving me home.

And to the wonderful Floridian oranges sent by the Igou family!

FEEDBACK FROM ARTHUR SABATINI

The following response was sent by Arthur Sabatini to my comments about the relationship between love and revolutionary war.

> Your diaries are extraordinary. I am amazed at the depth and lucidity of what you are writing. I have little to say about the treatment and medical/health issues, which you seem to be on top of. However, your decision to affirm Love is powerful, real and meaningful and I just want to be with you on that. Like music, poetry, friendship and imagination, love is one of the ways of being human that has been disabused and ignored by the limited worldview of the contemporary world. Worse, it has been

undermined by the discourses of romanticism, psychology and subsumed by religion, when it really belongs with poets (and I mean the poetry in everyone). To the degree that there is a history of love, it is, complexly, a way of being that is at once actual, defiant, selfless. To love, like the freest music in performance, is open-ended and conversant. It is aware of itself and desires engagement with others to continue creatively. It is a test of the self and the otherness of the self and being itself. (The Knights, warriors of their time, were expected to be able to fight, write poetry and pursue love). True lovers, as Octavio Paz, pointed out somewhere, are a threat to the State because they value life and the State is consumed with power and control. The connections between love and imagination are well known. And music. Well... of course.

The Russian thinker Mikhail Bakhtin wrote a book about laughter (another key subject) said, "Certain essential elements of the world are accessible only through laughter." He could have said, "Certain essential elements of the world are accessible only through love." But, you know that.

ARTHUR SABATINI

DIARY 17: THE WAR CONTINUES

March 12, 2008

I finished combined chemo-radiation at the end of January 2008. After two to three weeks, I began to regain energy and many of the side effects (extreme fatigue, awful zits, diarrhea) began to subside. I started to practice my sax again daily, compose, and completed a new work "Every Time I Open My Mouth to Sing" commissioned by baritone vocalist Tom Buckner (written for him and myself on baritone sax) with text by Jayne Cortez. I also resumed my exercise workout and regular swimming. By early March, I felt very good.

During this time, I had regular blood tests, a CEA (cancer cell count) test, a PET/CT, and MRI scan. Today, March 12, 2008, I met with my surgeon, Dr. Antonio Picon, who reviewed all the tests with me. He told me the tests were excellent and that all indications seem to demonstrate that the chemo-radiation treatments were effective in reducing the size of both tumors. He discussed with me the next stage of the war: surgery to remove the bigger colorectal tumor, examination of the smaller pelvic tumor (and preparation to treat it possibly with injective radiation during the surgery) and the creation of an ileostomy (exterior bag to redirect my urine and fecal excretions). This operation will be March 27. It is not certain that interjection radiation will be done, but they are preparing for it in a special lead-encased room as I will become radioactive for a couple of days. Medical staff will have to wear special protective lead attire. Visitors will not be allowed until the isotopes are dissipated.

Many of you have been asking about visiting me in the hospital. The safest thing is to contact the colorectal surgery physicians assistant, Ms. Vicki Brooks, or my friend Ann T. Greene.

I will be in the hospital for seven to ten days (March 27 to April 3, 2008) at Beth Israel, First Avenue and Sixteenth Street, Manhattan. I will *not* have a phone. It is best you call either Ann or the physicians assistant to see if I'm still there and the visiting hours.

When I return home, I will not be able to lift anything heavy or exert myself. I will have difficulty for the first two to three weeks sitting up and walking. During the months of April and May, I will need whatever assistance all of you can give: coming over to go for a walk around the block, picking up groceries, cooking, and some cleaning. You can call me at my home phone or e-mail as to when you'd like to visit. During this time, I'll have to have regular doctor appointments and evaluate if I'll have more chemo-radiation treatments in June–July.

A special thanks to Joyce Gibney for sending me wonderful health information and for the cod liver oil. Continued thanks to Annetta and Woody Igou for the delicious and nutritious Florida oranges.

DIARY 18: HELL IS A MANSION OF MANY ROOMS

April 26, 2008

Note from Ann, May 13, 2008: This long-overdue transmission contains a diary entry notable for its humor and candor. For Fred, the last few months have been filled with struggles and achievements, both physical and spiritual. Yet during that time he wrote moving tributes to colleagues Raul Salinas and Max Roach that are a joy to read.

Also attached are some food guidelines and general advice from Flora Hoffman, Fred's sister. Some of you have already received this in mid-April, but I wanted to make sure everyone who was cooking for Fred had it. By now, Fred's diet has expanded to include more foods, but this information is still useful when planning meals.

Special thanks to the friends who have called and visited Fred these past few weeks since his release from Beth Israel in April. Kokua, all— your practical and loving help is a gift for all warriors. In appreciation,

ANN

TO REACH JOURNEY'S END, I RETURN TO HELL

March 25 to April 25, 2008

In the fall of 2007, after two colonoscopies and MRI and PT/CT scans, it was confirmed that the colorectal tumor had returned, and there was possibility that another tumor had grown in my pelvic area. It was also absolutely clear that the first-line industry chemotherapy for stage 3b colon cancer, FOLFOX, was completely ineffective in my case.

I was given one in four chances (25 percent) of living by my new oncologist, Dr. Peter Kozuch. Very few studies and reports were available for my unique and dangerous condition. In consultation with Dr. Kenneth Hu, radiation oncologist at Beth Israel Medical Center, a plan was devised in which I would have simultaneous daily radiation treatments in conjunction with daily chemotherapy at home via pills and weekly infusions in the hospital's chemo suite. This would happen for six weeks from mid-December to the end of January 2008. My previous two cancer war diary entries detailed that journey through hell.

In the two months I had to recover from that trip to hell, I spent the first two weeks sleeping and restoring my energy. Then I embarked upon a daily regimen of alternating between basic isometrics and hand-to-hand combat training outdoors in the park and swimming at the city pool. I also practiced the saxophone daily, increasing my chi energy through the horn. I gained weight. I continued with supplements of vitamin C, iron, calcium, selenium, vitamin D, omega-3 fatty acid, and multivitamins. I also ate a banana a day for added potassium and at least one delicious juicy Florida orange sent by the Igou family in Orlando. (During that past radio-chemo treatment, my blood cell counts with regard to potassium, magnesium, and iron had dropped, hence the need for those particular supplements.

I returned for a second surgery on March 25, 2008, at 11:00 AM. I had been through this before, and I felt strong, prepared, knowledgeable of what to expect, and how to deal. My sister Dr. Florence Houn met me at the admitting area, and to my utmost surprise, my longtime friend and musical comrade, the great Dr. Hafez Modirzadeh, was also there. He had read an earlier e-mail that stated my admitting time was 9:00 AM, so he had been sitting in the waiting area for two hours. He couldn't stay very long and gave me loving words of support and a strong hug.

At about 1:00 PM I was put under anesthesia and went to sleep.

I am told that the surgery took eight hours. The result in the opinion of the surgeon, Dr. Antonio Picon, was very positive and encouraging. What was thought to be a second tumor in my pelvis turned out to be benign. The colorectal tumor was successfully removed with no signs of spread or metastases to vital organs. I was transferred to the intensive care unit (ICU). When I woke up, and I'm not sure what time it was the next day; I was still groggy and barely able to open my eyes but was lovingly greeted by my sister, my dearest friends Gwen Mok and her husband Rick, and then they were soon joined by Hafez. Hafez stood up over me and began to extemporize a lecture on man and music. The hospital staff and Florence had never seen or heard such a thing happen before. Professor Modirzadeh, the most innovative music theorist of our era and a titanic saxophonist, espoused on and on. While I wasn't able to pay attention or stay awake, his melodious voice helped me rest and put me to sleep! I don't know how long he lectured for. But it had the effect of giving me peace.

My sister informed me that I would experience a gradation of quality from the nursing staff during my hospital stay. The ICU nurses were the top shelf. The only problem was the constant noise and talking in a pretty open area (no real private rooms where doors could be closed). I was constantly awakened by the noise and bustle there. I also was suffering from sinus congestion and need to rinse my nostrils without blowing too hard and risking tearing my newly sewn stomach. I also craved cool water and was given ice chips, which were very comforting and soothing to me. I later craved cold apple juice, but I overdid it, and it distended my belly. I had to then be told to stay off of it, which I did.

Ann Greene, Mark O'Ferrall, and Mike Surdej came by as well to look in on me. To the surprise of the ICU staff, I got myself up and out of bed pretty easily. I had learned how to do it the first time I had surgery by shifting my body weight to my legs and letting them serve as weighted leverage to drop to the ground and with my upper body strength (which I had worked on before surgery with increasing numbers of front and back chin-ups and push ups), push my body erect. I sat in a chair for a couple of hours, very tired and groggy but enjoying everyone's company.

After two days, I was downgraded to standard recovery in a room on the tenth floor. And I then experienced the unevenness of nursing professionalism. Some nurses were perfunctory, slackers, others were gems, in particular two personal care attendants (PCAs): Jeannie and Pamela. They were very caring and attentive, doing whatever I needed and anticipating my care needs. After I was discharged, I wrote a letter to Beth Israel commending these two PCAs and requesting their promotion.

While in the recovery room, many visitors came by: Ann and Mark regularly, Howard Stokar and Charles Wuorinen, Joe Russoto, Monika H., Taylor Ho Bynum, and Abraham Gomez-Delgado; and if I forgot to mention others, I apologize, but I was seriously experiencing the worst of sleep deprivation.

Sleeping for the next six days was nearly impossible, with interruptions from tests and monitoring that had to be done, but the worst was the constant need to empty my ileostomy bag that now was attached to my upper intestines and sticking out of my stomach to the right of my belly button. My friend, Dr. Stephanie Athey, a specialist in torture, described what I underwent as what victims of torture experience from sleep deprivation.

My catheter was removed, and I had to pee within twelve hours or risk infection. I couldn't pee, and the nurse was getting very frustrated with me, constantly asking me while I was trying to sleep, "Have you gone pee pee? Have you gone pee pee?" I could tell the task of replacing the catheter was something nurses didn't like or want to do. Since I didn't "go pee pee," it was put back in, though I didn't have too much pain. (All my extensions such as the ileostomy bag, the catheter, and other tubings were all initially installed when I was under anesthesia.) I have to commend the seriousness given by Beth Israel to pain management. A morphine subcutaneous port was installed during surgery at the base of my spine, so I was morphined for the first few days, and pain was minimal. Well, I did pee pee once the catheter was reinstalled. After a while, the catheter was once again removed, and I had to try to go pee pee without it. Fortunately, as the twelve-hour mark was approaching, I managed to urinate on my own and filled the container. A shout of joy resonated through the recovery room corridor, as the new nurse was relieved, and she wouldn't have to reinstall the catheter.

This second surgery recovery has had a lot less pain or difficulty for me in being mobile (e.g., getting out of bed and walking around). But it has been worse in terms of intense grogginess and fatigue due to sleep deprivation. I had to argue with a night nurse to simply close the door and turn off the lights after she finished her checkups. She was simply too unwilling to simply be mindful about doing that in order for myself and the other patient I shared the room with to get some sleep. The other patient was too timid, but I got him to voice his wanting to have the door closed and lights off, so she did it. Whew, the simple battles and fights that a patient must wage to get rest and peace.

After six days, after I proved I could pee on my own, learned how to empty and change the ileostomy bag, and ingest a small portion of solid food, I was discharged. I had brought a bag of books and CDs, all of which I was too tired and exhausted to get to during my stay.

Joanne Maffia, my composition student, pushed my wheelchair, while Ann Greene carried my bags, and I was driven home by Mark O'Ferrall. I couldn't wait to get to my apartment. Ahhh, the peace and quiet and warmth of my place. I fell into bed and to sleep immediately. Ann was so kind and helpful as to pick up beverages for me, prepare my ileostomy bags and other basic chores to make sure I could have a smooth transition back to my home.

I hadn't encountered these postsurgery experiences the first time that I now faced:

The lack of sleep for twelve days. Even at home, the new challenge of the ileostomy bag enslaved me to its schedule of every 1.5 to 3 hours of getting up and emptying it. I had to be fully awake, use both hands, or I'd be careless and the feces would splash and make a mess, causing me to be angry and even more frustrated. I didn't have an appetite, had lost twenty-seven pounds. I needed to eat, I understood this. But eat what? For the first two and a half weeks, I was struggling to figure out what I could stomach. For the first week or so, it was mostly liquids: Jell-O, juices, soup, cheese and crackers, bread and butter. I couldn't handle fiber, certainly not nuts, raw fruits, and vegetables were impossible.

The love of my life, Melanie, stayed with me for a few days and prepared small meals at my request. It was hard for her as my constant getting up in the night interrupted her sleep. She could feel my misery and difficulties and gave me her unconditional love.

My youngest sister Flora and my two nieces overlapped with Mel's stay. They were fun to be with and drew me lovely pictures, which I have hanging on my apartment door. The loving warmth they gave me helped me fight the depression that would soon overwhelm me after they left.

I soon realized that I was suffering from combat fatigue, war weariness, and that depression was beginning for me. The sleep debt was enormous, and it demanded repayment, which I couldn't do. I began to lose it. There was a point, and torture victims are driven to this state of complete breakdown of self and identity, that I lost/forget who I am. After twelve-plus days of barely any sleep, I was a broken man, unable to gather together a sense of who I am. I cried and cried. I had to read essays people like Peggy Choy, Bill Mullen, Ruth Margraff, Diane Fujino, and others wrote about me for a forthcoming book about my work edited by Dr. Roger Buckley in order to remind myself of who I am and to regain my sense of self. Bill had mentioned in his essay for almost two years I have been fighting this war and most of the time I have been in bed. Only about seven months were good, and I could return to the activity I had before the war began. Without intellectual and creative stimulation and activity, I am cut off from the energy that makes me who I am. But this new phase of the war, I was completely drained of energy, unlike the first postsurgery, where energy more quickly returned to me, and I could socialize, talk to people on the phone, write my cancer war diary, make plans, go out for meals with people, etc.

This time, I was bone-drained tired, energyless. Last time I had lost twelve pounds; this time I lost more than double that amount of weight. I could barely eat; I no longer enjoyed food. *And if the next intimate details are too personal for you, skip forward two paragraphs.*

And worse, I felt I had lost my manhood. I still cannot have an erection or ejaculate. My love Melanie tells me she thinks I'm the sexiest man still, even cut up with holes in my stomach and a shit collecting bag sticking from it. I am in a constant stupor, and I feel stupid, the simplest life activities being a source of anger and frustration.

The ileostomy bag, I felt, was my enemy; I hated it and at times wanted to rip it from me like in the hospital in 2006 when the waste evacuation tube from my stomach through my esophagus through my nostril was clogging my breathing; I simply tore out the meter long tube and threw it away from me. It is the desperation and anger that drives me to violence, such as taking a knife and cutting off one's own body part in a total explosion of irrationality. I have deliberately cut myself before, to drain infections. I don't fear pain or hurt, but sleep deprivation, loss of self, produce a misery of wallowing, engulfing hopelessness that for the first time in my life, I could truly understand why people commit suicide. The toll, the debt, they realize, is too much and can never be repaid. We want an end, a finality. I will never ever forget this state I was in as a secret chamber of darkness and despair that I don't ever again want to open the door to, much less enter that room.

But Peggy Choy, my *kokua*, gave some sublime Buddhist teaching. She said to me, "Fred, learn to love your bag." It changed my perspective and attitude, revolutionized me.

I have very little energy to even talk to people. Before I looked forward to getting out and walking (though the weather was much warmer then in September of 2006 with Indian summer). The prolonged winter we've had, the rain, dampness, and cold, have increased the weariness and weakness I have. When the days are sunny and warm, I feel better. I gradually get stronger daily, energy returning to me in incremental amounts. I am back to eating very small portions of solid foods, most everything, though nothing too fibrous, especially no nuts, and still on the mild side, though Abraham Gomez-Delgado brought over some delicious Puerto Rican rice and beans and I added some Tabasco sauce. I could both handle it and enjoyed it *caliente*.

By week 3's end of postsurgery, I started to sleep better, in three-hour cycles. I hesitated to take Benadryl as a sleep inducement, but finally did, but its helpfulness was minor. Now I get up once or twice during the night to pee and to empty the bag, but can usually fall asleep again, and if not, I watch a movie or check e-mails, and when I get tired, I just go to bed to return to sleep.

The weariness has reduced my interest in socializing with people and my friends, and I feel miserable about this. I love all of you so dearly. You are all giving, generous, compassionate, and brilliant people; and I welcome the laughs, the stories, the ideas, the sunshine you all convey and impart, but there are times I can barely stay awake or even have the energy to explain what I need or want done when you offer to come over and help. Rest and the chance to sleep has become the center of my existence for now. Please understand. I will need your love, attention, help, and stimulation soon, more than ever as I have begun the worse part of this journey in my return to hell.

THE RETURN TO HELL AGAIN, BEFORE A LIFE ANEW

On April 25, 2008, I started up again on a third round of chemo. Daily for fourteen days, once a week in the hospital (Fridays) for infusions in twenty-one-day cycles, with the third week off the daily chemo, but still the once-a-week in-hospital treatment. Mike Surdej was so lovingly kind and helpful to pick me up with his car at 8:00 AM, take me to the hospital, stay with me for four and a half hours, drive me home. I was really wasted. I couldn't even give Mike a conversation. It is worse than before because the two previous chemo treatments, even the last one that was combined with daily radiation, I had weeks and months to recover and was in optimum conditioning. I am just four weeks out of surgery, still healing and recovering from that, compounded with sleep deprivation, much smaller food intake, that my body is not as strong as I need it to be to face another twelve weeks of chemo. Dr. Kozuch says to me, "You know the drill, all the same side effect a as before—zits exploding, diarrhea, nausea, exhaustion, and fatigue. You faced a lot, no, too much, but there is light at the end of the tunnel. We are going to go for cure. Hopefully, in a few months after this all ends, it'll just be a distant bad memory." This is all cause for a lot of hope, far from what he told me in fall 2007 of the one in four chances of living. I have to reaffirm this goal into my entire being.

I am truly wasted now. I hope all of you can be *kokua*. From the native Hawaiian culture, introduced to me by brother Richard Hamasaki of Kaneohe, Oahu, a *kokua* is someone who gives help, aid, assistance, relief, a comforter, a benefactor, a "partner in crime," but in a deeply spiritual sense, akin to the Judeo-Christian concept of a guardian angel, someone who stands guard, watchful, vigilant, caring, protective, helpful, who stands by you in the most terrible and worst of times. In Klingon mythology, an entity who travels with a slain warrior on the River Styx to fight off the predators and demons who seek to ravage and claim the heart and soul of the warrior at his/her weakest moment. I need all of you to be such beings, *kokua*, for this one more journey back to hell and through the gauntlet of ravages so that I may come to a life anew, changed forever, fighting forever.

Postscript addendum: Memorials to Max Roach and Raul Salinas.

Below are two essays I wrote as praise tributes to fallen warrior-comrades who have been mentors, supporters, and exemplars to me.

Published in Volume 8 Number 1 issue of 2008 *Black Renaissance Noire*:

Max Roach
Rest in Peace
January 10, 1924–August 15, 2007

ALL PRAISE DUE TO MAX ROACH: With his *Passing the Reign of the Regurgitators Has Begun*

Max Roach, heralded as "the greatest jazz drummer of all time," passed away on August 15, 2007. With his death, jazz died. An era has come to an end for a music that was once arguably the revolutionary new music of the twentieth century: a music that embraced the greatness of improvisation, a supreme technical mastery fueled by the profoundest commitment to human liberation.

Both the music and the great artists who expressed these energies and characteristics emerged and developed from an intrinsic communal context. At Max's public memorial service at Riverside Church this past August, close friend pianist Randy Weston, himself now an elder, told the story how when he was a youth he would go over to Max's Brooklyn home regularly and sit for hours listening to the conversations between Max, Miles Davis, Thelonius Monk, and so many of the great artists, as well as listening to rehearsals that served as community laboratories in which the most advanced ideas were being developed for twentieth-century music.

All of that is gone. Today's young musicians go to colleges and universities for their music training, where they receive tremendous amounts of technical training, and many of them are technical prodigies and wunderkinds. However, they have no imagination and, worse, no commitment to liberation. In today's jazz, they reign supreme. Today is the Reign of the Regurgitators.

These Regurgitators are the human equivalent to computer sampling. They are like biological iPods who can play very convincingly styles from the past, but they have no styles of their own.

Jazz may now be truly dead. The once-revolutionary music for the planet is now a regurgitated artifact.

Max Roach knew this even as early as the late 1970s when he realized two things:

First, he could no longer have a band of his peers whose desire to make music embodied improvisation and liberation as its supreme mission.

And second, his former peers (who were the great innovators of the 1940s and 1950s), for one reason or another, while perhaps still committed to liberation, could no longer be innovative. Perhaps they were preoccupied with continuing a jazz career in an industry that rewarded the glory of ol' chestnuts and rebuked "the new thing." Perhaps some had become feeble and weak from years of hardship and struggle, such as Thelonius Monk. Others had become commercially acquisitive. And still others, such as Dizzy Gillespie and Sonny Rollins, while still commanding players, no longer sought radical innovation, becoming complacent in their commanding competence.

Only one musician seemed to continually defy complacency and commercial predictability (of either relying upon the "ol' chestnuts" or "crossing over" into more mass-marketed commercial forms): Max Roach. Max, while keeping his quartet, however, refocused his energies on duets with major innovators of his time, musicians and artists of other disciplines who would challenge the parameters of jazz conception and performance. These included the following: Anthony Braxton, Cecil Taylor, Fab 5 Freddy, theater director George Ferencz, Amiri Baraka, Archie Shepp, the Kodo Drummers of Sato Island/Japan, dancer/choreographer Bill T. Jones, and Dianne MacIntyre, to forming the all-percussion ensemble, M'Boom, and so many other collaborations.

The jazz band of today has become a hierarchal star vehicle and not the kind of unit that constantly purveys a revolutionary tradition, uniting innovators collectively seeking new musical terrain and new energies toward expressive liberation. Perhaps the jazz band as we know it today has become exhausted as a vehicle for creative formulation and instead become entertainment spectacle for a sanitized past nostalgia. The point is not to debate or argue for which period of jazz is more advanced than others, but to transcend and transform tradition. The revolutionary character of twentieth-century jazz that the reigning canon constructionists and gatekeepers Wynton Marsalis, Stanley Crouch, and Albert Murray fail to recognize, and, more heinously, deny is the music's dialectic: innovation and liberation are mutual, interdependent sides of the same coin. Both the musical and sociocultural theory and practice of jazz is the interdependency and inextricability of improvisation/innovation and liberation.

Not coincidentally, there is a concomitant lack of innovative development in African American political theory and practice, hence the movement and the music have fallen into a rut of regurgitation.

Max realized even as early as the 1970s that the conventional jazz band wasn't a sufficient-enough vehicle to fire his radical imagination, to inspire his expressive transcendence, and assert cultural transformation. The music industry is incapable of and inimical toward any formations that deviate from the star-leader-with-side-persons model of a band. The deeper question, one that Max struggled with and was unable to solve, is the economics (making money) with forms that do not have a place or position in the current music marketplace. That's a tall order to ask or expect artists to figure out: the question of building a new economic apparatus, though Max understood that such an effort would have to utilize nonjazz institutions. Artistic innovation has always preceded institutional and economic change, the latter having to be found or made to service the former. For example, the after-hours venues in the 1940s were the sites of incubation for what has come to be called bebop. In the 1960s, community settings were the sites for the new music experiments. In the 1970s, Lower Manhattan lofts were the sites for the so-called loft jazz endeavors. Those long hours of rehearsing and conversation need places for incubation and venues before the public that provide some recompense. Extramusical collaborations between artists and organizers and entrepreneurs are essential to realizing anything that asserts to be truly alternative.

Even in the last several years of his life, with the growing affliction of Alzheimer's disease, Max continued to quest for the new, albeit too weak, results quite possibly due to the severe debilitations wrought on by the disease. While a small handful of musicians from Max's emergent era of the bebop revolution are still actively performing today, none embody the tremendous leadership that Max exerted, both as an irrepressible innovator and liberation fighter. With the passing of Max Roach, the last leading stalwart opposition to the Reign of the Regurgitators is gone. When an art form becomes more preoccupied with the past and finer degrees of interpretations of that past, it truly has become a museum artifact. But inevitably, and inexorably, rebellion and resistance will foment, most likely from communities and sites most marginalized and maligned, uncontaminated by the sterility and sanitization that is engendered by the salacious desire to support the status quo.

SPEECH GIVEN APRIL 18, 2008, AT THE BRECHT FORUM, NYC

Raul Salinas, born March 17, 1934, passed on February 14, 2008, after years of struggle with a myriad of medical maledictions rooted in growing up under severe conditions of oppression in the oppressed Indio-Xicano nation of Atzlan, from fifteen years of incarceration, most of which was spent in the supermax hellholes of America's prisons, all of which produced years of habits that neglected the importance of nutrition, proper hydration, and clean living.

I met Raul in the early 1990s at an annual multicultural literary festival organized by the Guadalupe Cultural Center of San Antonio, Texas, when black arts poet Kalamu ya Salaam and I performed there in our Afro Asian Arts Dialogue duet of Kalamu blowing poetry and I reciting the baritone sax. Raul came up to us and introduced himself and gave us a personally signed copy of one of his poetry chapbooks. It wasn't until about a half decade later, after my frequent travels to Austin, Texas, where Raul lived and worked, after listening to his baritone profundo voice on several CD recordings he had made that that sound of his voice, plus of course his revolutionary words, inspired me to reach out to him to collaborate. We began Caliente! Circle Around the Sun, which soon added Boriqua-Gitano poetess extraordinaire Magdalena Gomez, whom I also collaborate with separately. In the few years we were a poetry-music unit, we performed on both coasts and in Minnesota upon the support of Professors Louis Mendoza (Raul's friend and principal biographer at the University of Minnesota in Minneapolis) and Peter Rachleff, labor scholar and activist at MacAlester College in St. Paul.

Raul grew up poor in the ghettos of the massive oppressed brown communities of Texas, a cultural rebel and what today we might describe as "gang banger" and street person. He partied hard and began his consumption of cigarettes and alcohol. He was arrested and convicted on a marijuana possession, but typical of so many oppressed youth, lacking money and status that would avail to oneself greater dispensation in the legal system, the state basically locked him up and threw away the key. He was expected to rot in jail for the rest of his life. But as Raul tells it in his Louis Mendoza—edited collection, *raulsalinas and the Jail Machine: My Pen Is My Weapon* (University of Texas Press, 2006), he was saved from despair and cynicism, and indeed transformed, while in prison by the power of jazz music. He began to write music and recording reviews and commentaries, which developed into his own creative verse and jazz poetic style. The outside world began to take note of his growing literary output.

And then the revolutionary 1960s hit hard, and even America's most desolate and isolated corners, such as its prisons, felt this tsunami of revolt. Raul became of one America's leading prison intellectuals and revolutionaries. His writings became important communiqués to the outside world about the horrid conditions behind the walls and the growing struggles by prisoners themselves to challenge what has now come to be called "the prison industrial complex." While in prison, Raul wrote a penetrating analysis and commentary, *Un Trip Through the Mind Jail and Otras Excursions*, which has since become a classic. It is a must-read for all activists in its analysis and insights about prisons as institutions of repression, social control, and colonization/national oppression.

During the late 1960s, a group of socially conscious professors and students at the University of Washington–Seattle took up the cause of gaining the release of Raul. After years of steadfast diligence and dedication, Raul Salinas was gained his freedom in 1972, having served fifteen years of his youth incarcerated, eleven of those years in some of America's most brutal prisons.

Raul immediately plunged himself into the revolutionary movements of the day. He founded the Leonard Peltier Defense Committee, was active in the founding of the American Indian Movement, in the Marxist-Leninist party-building movement, a major figure in revolutionary cultural work especially as a poet, Native American and Xicano liberation (he has been a vanguard unity builder of an Indigenous-Chicano identity), and represented a multiplicity of movements and struggles at international conferences and gatherings across the globe, all the while being rooted in his local community of Austin's east side. There, he founded Red Salmon Press and the independent bookstore Resistencia. While it is now trendy to speak of "intersectionality" in academic circles, Raul, like so many of us, could never be narrowly pigeonholed in his revolutionary politics: he was Indio-Xicano liberation fighter, cultural worker-poet, communist, hipster, jazz lover and scholar, and so on. He not only embodied the confluence of all these movements, but he was also a leading figure in all of them as well.

One of the last cultural productions was our collaborative CD, *Red Arc*. Throughout his years, Raul has always been a hipster; indeed, he moved among the Beat poets, but like so much of American historical accounts, he and the other oppressed nationality proponents have been largely ignored in most white supremacist accounting of American cultural movements, both mainstream and counterculture. Only LeRoi Jones is given recognition, while other oppressed nationality jazz poets of the Beat era, such as the Japanese American Lawson Fusao Inada, the late African-mixed heritage Bob Kaufman, and others, are ignored. What makes for a jazz poet? Let's listen to an example from the CD so you can hear the Lester Young–like coolness, the Thelonious Monk–like angularity, the interactivity and intrinsic improvisational primacy, and existentiality of expression.

DIARY 19: BEYOND THE BEYOND, WHEN YOU CANNOT GO BACK, YOU CAN ONLY GO FORWARD

April 26 to June 9, 2008

I began my third round of chemotherapy on April 25, 2008, which will go until July 12, 2008. My main side effects are zits, fatigue, some nausea, jitters, and cramping during my intravenous chemo sessions at the hospital, for which medications have helped alleviate. After the chemo is done, I will have surgery again to remove the ileostomy bag and reconnect my insides, and need to heal and recover.

I am hoping to be well enough to begin my artist in residency at the University of Wisconsin–Madison beginning the last few days of August and going to mid-December. I'll be teaching a course titled Revolutionary Afro Asian Performance and Spoken Word, working with students to develop innovative text and to perform them based upon the forms and traditions primarily emanating from the African and Asian diasporas. I will use a methodology for teaching from the black arts movement (integrating theory and practice, with performance as primary; collective accountability in self-education; mutual criticism/self-criticism; experimentalism toward innovation; inspiring and catalyzing the masses; etc.).

Because chemo kills all cells, both good and bad, the healing of my surgical wound has been slowed down. With the beginning of this chemo round, I experienced greater and prolonged pain, greater restriction in my activity and recovery. Recently, my oncologist, Dr. Kozuch, decided to have me off all chemo for one week and off two chemo drugs for two weeks to help the cellular regeneration. This period allowed me to gain greater strength, energy, and activity. The full chemo regimen was resumed on June 6.

During this hiatus off chemo, my life energy returned. My voice started to sound like the familiar Fred Ho. I was able to practice my saxophone again and have continued to do so every day, at the break of dawn for approximately an hour a day. I was happy to find that I hadn't lost very much in my playing. I still am unable to exercise except by taking walks. Until I feel confidant that my stomach wound has fully healed, I do not want to risk tearing it especially when the chemo has delayed the cellular restitution.

I have used my time in hell and the moments of lucidity and energy. I have had to begin some deep philosophical pondering on my future and how I should continue to live life either cancer free or should the cancer not be beaten, how to live the rest of my days on this planet. I share with you below this vision quest.

THE DEATH OF THE OLD FRED HO AND THE BEGINNING OF THE NEW FRED HO

I have resolved that I cannot return to the carcinogenic life I once had. Scientists continually debate whether colorectal cancer can be attributable to any direct causes, such as types of foods and the ways they are prepared, lifestyle, etc., with the only generally acceptable attribution being heredity. But in my heart and soul, I believe that in my case, eating high-temperature cooked foods (broiled, grilled, deep fried), combined with high-fat foods (e.g., ice cream) is something I am not willing to return to anymore. I haven't resolved to become vegan, macrobiotic, or a lacto-ovo vegetarian; but I will make the concentration of my diet to be primarily raw foods, with a significant reduction in animal-source fats and proteins. Now daily I eat all kinds of green leafy vegetables, especially different kinds of spinach and salad greens. *I thank the inspiration of Stephanie Hughley and others for the personal, societal, and planetary benefits of a raw and plant-based diet.*

But the main source of toxicity for me has been the music/arts business. I have resolved that I will not return. I will continue to create and perform music and my operas (what were once referred to as my projects—multimedia vision quests, martial arts ballets/music/theater epics, etc.). But I will figure out how to pay my artists, gather resources to produce my work in all media (print, performance, digital), earn a little bit for myself (toward realizing my personal bucket list below), have resources for the Fred Ho Foundation for when I do kick the bucket, and hopefully leave some kind of revolutionary legacy.

What does it mean "not to return to the music/arts business"? I am completely *off* the treadmill of career, gig solicitation, hustling, self-promotion, networking, etc. It is the competition and comparison inherent in this business that I believe contributed to my being vulnerable to cancer, the toxicity of frustration, anger, etc., that are all too pervasive in the fight to be the artist that I am. I will *not* return to any of this.

I have in many ways been for the past nearly three decades a maverick and done things completely contrary to the mainstream music business. For example, in 1987, I swore never to play another club in America for these reasons: clubs exploit artists, clubs exploit audiences, clubs are carcinogenic environments. I kept this vow and found totally new venues such as Asian American student clubs, supportive/sympathetic college professors, galleries, cultural centers and presenting institutions, festivals that aren't "jazz"-oriented, etc.

I embarked upon self-producing big experimental shows (such as my operas, "martial arts," ballets, etc.), often at devastating financial losses to myself (e.g., over seven years, I expended $70,000 of my own money on furthering *Voice of the Dragon: Once Upon a Time in Chinese America . . .*), always believing in my work and my artistic collaborators, which eventually culminated in catapulting me onto a bigger stage of recognition and reward far beyond big-name jazz artists (e.g., the big names play the three-hundred-seat theater while my show will play to two sold out shows at the two-thousand-seat theater).

I never got married, never had children—my mantra was "If it came to paying my artists or feeding my kids, my kids would starve."

I downsized my life, contrary to the American dream of bigger homes, bigger cars (never owned one my entire life and never intend to own one!), bigger waistlines, more and more, accumulate. In 2000, I sold 70 percent of my material belongings, including a mammoth duplex loft in yuppie-infested Park Slope, bought a significantly cheaper place, was the general contractor, and designed and led the ten-week renovations on my present domicile. My expenses significantly dropped enabling me to be completely debt-free forever, have a secure retirement should I chose to retire immediately, and to do whatever I want, even at financial loss to myself (though not for an indefinite period of time), liberating me to make my choices solely based on the following reason for why I believe I was put on this planet:

> To make the music/art and promote the politics for which *no one else can or will do*. To take on the most difficult, challenging, but the most necessary work. These are reflected in my bucket list below as well.

Marty Khan pointed out to me, to paraphrase, Fred, all your life, you've done things differently and against the tide. We are exploring the path of exiting the worn and dying path of finding booking agents, hustling and scrambling for gigs, piecing together tours, dealing with declining record distribution and sales, and all the moribund means, methods, and manifestations of a music-arts industry controlled by gatekeepers who have little or no concern or passion for the innovative, transgressive, and liberating.

Personally, I am beginning the journey to eliminate all *ego*. Even if it comes with extreme hostility and malignancy, I will seek and embrace the smallest grain of truth. I seek no gain or accumulation of anything except experience, wisdom, and love. I will make integrity and love the foundation of all of my interactions and exchanges.

In my previous diary entry in my eulogy to Max Roach, I asserted that "jazz is dead." In matters of artistry and aesthetics, my music will no longer reference past forms and "the tradition" but *become an aesthetic of being beyond the beyond*. I want the future years of my sound, my saxophone playing, my composing to go far beyond what I've done, to no longer reference that which I've done already, but embark upon the beyond. I will only do commissions for *those who seek me out*. I will no longer solicit existing configurations. Rather than seek to enter, be accepted by the mainstream, the establishment, the conventional, I will do what I do and accept any and all those who come to me because of what I stand for, and who can deal with me as I am, and desire that energy and being, who seek me as a friend, artist and fellow traveler, as common adventurers who boldly seek the beyond as well.

(Sun Ra has influenced the above, though I am a Luddite and not a technology fetishist. For me, technology is human creative labor, not simply machines, and tools need not be electromagnetic generating, but utilize other energies.)

A NEW WAY TO MAKE LOVE

I met with urologist Dr. Aaron Grotas about my sexual dysfunction. He explained that one inadvertent consequence of the last surgery may have been nerve damage from the movement and redirection of my internals. While I am able to have an erection, I cannot ejaculate. He believes that in a year's time, this function may return. However, if within a year, it does not, it will most likely never return.

The cost of the cancer war has been a lot of physical loss (the latest being the possibly permanent loss of ejaculation). But I accept the challenge to create a male nonphallocentric way to make love. And the love of my life, my Mellow Warrior, will accompany me on this journey of mutual sensual pleasure beyond the ejaculatory orgasm. Instead of an outer-directed orgasm, to attain an inner-inspired orgasm.

The cancer war taught me new ways of breathing and how to approach life at the cellular level. It has given me a new way to play the saxophone, for example. I embrace the *beyond*ness: to figure out a new way to live beyond what physical losses and limitations have occurred, to be open to discovery, revelation, rejuvenation, and revolutionary transcendence and transformation. When you cannot go back, then you can only go forward.

MY BUCKET LIST (SO FAR)

1. To snorkel in the open ocean with orcas, blue whales, and sperm whales;
2. To teach and share what I've learned on this planet;
3. To help make a revolution without egotism and militarism;
4. To help generate artist-empowered new media and ways of expression and dissemination that supersedes any system of "gatekeeping": in other words, in the profound words of Peggy Choy, to build "the gateless gate" (excellence and imagination without stratification).

THE BEAUTIFUL OUTPOURING

Many people were moved and inspired by my last diary entry and gave both heartfelt missives and all kinds of assistance. I'd like to share some of these responses and also thank the generosity of my beloved kokuas (warrior angels-protectors).

From Beverly Naidus, Vachon Island, Washington:

Dearest Fred,

We think of you often, and have been for many, many months keeping you in our hearts. You, of course, are turning this journey into hell into a teaching for all of us. We greatly admire your gift for doing this, and are very grateful to have you, even from afar, in our lives.

With much love,

BEVERLY

Her husband, Bob Spivey, also sent this message:

Fred,

What an incredibly honest, moving, and powerful diary entry. All the gifts and energies you have brought together in the struggle against capitalism—the cancer of social life—you have now mobilized against a very non-metaphorical cancer: music, love, connection, commitment, directly naming truth, physical knowledge and prowess, keen yet poetic intellect, humor, and now a profound openness to blessings of all kinds. Also the tribute to Max Roach is among the very best writing on jazz I have come across. I think of you in reading Legacy to Liberation on the need for clear revolutionary ideology, disciplined political strategy, and new political organization, and also when I sit in our kitchen and read the Sheroes calendar. I have warm memories of seeing you at Beverly's presentation at Bluestockings, and of the Chinese restaurant below ground you took us to later that, among other things, cured our son Sam's stomach problems that had been lasting for days. May you find special nourishment now in your underground struggle.

I see people's bags every other day in my work now, and sometimes help clean them. You're no less of a warrior with a bag, maybe more.

BOB SPIVEY

From my good snorkeling buddy, Woody Igou in Orlando, Florida:

Dear Fred:

I just read your latest diary entry, which was forwarded. You are quite brave and profound (indeed your diary is a De Profundis of its time). It strikes me that your life makes a statement about us all. Most of us, having gone through life with vast compromises from our youthful ideals, face our mortality with a different set of eyes than you do. We would say to ourselves in your situation—*now* I know the value of life! *Now* if I can get past this ordeal, I will live my life to the fullest, love life and live my ideals.

In your case - you <u>did</u> live your life that way, prior to and without the cleansing hand of illness. You had little to change on the big issues of life.

The mind set and discipline that you took <u>into</u> this battle is the mind set that usually only survivors possess <u>after</u> the fact. That is what will save you.

Yours with love,

WOODY

And finally, from brother Richard Hamasaki and his family (my *ohana*—Hawaiian for "family") of Kaneohe, Hawaii:

Dear Brother Fred:

Hope this e-mail finds you in good spirits and increasing strength!

Several weeks ago, I had a dream. You had finished tapping on your computer keyboard your last few words from your cancer diary and then you reached over and switched on a video.

In between bouts of sleep and darkness, grainy, digital video images revealed you working, composing tunes to words from your cancer diaries—short pieces—like songs—and they were being sung. Some were a cappella; some had a four-piece behind it; others had choruses, some harmonious, others cacophonic yet like the dove with mynah bird, so different (cooing versus grunting, gritty, throatiness of mynah in tonal/atonal voicings).

They were about your hellish journeys, abject depression, thirst, discomfort, pain, loneliness, but also honored caregivers as well as kokua and devotees of healing; of musicians who were healer revolutionaries; some tunes included words of advice– about getting enough sleep(!) and what to do when dealing with health care, bad nurses, open doors, glaring lights, chilled, metallic rooms, a sense of humor and irony prevailed.

They were short pieces, but why short? and why ditties, and why so much like bird song?

Well, when I woke up, it was still quite dark, but I as I heard the first tunes from birds outside our window singing in the bushes and trees, I then remembered your diaries; I switched on my night light and reread your diaries like poetry:

The prolonged winter we've had
the rain,
the dampness and cold
have increased the weariness
and weakness I have . . .

Abraham Gomes-Delgado
brought over some delicious
Puerto Rican rice and beans
and I added some Tabasco sauce
I could handle it
and enjoyed it
caliente . . .

Please understand
I will need your love
attention, help and stimulation soon,
more than ever
as I beg[i]n the worse

. . . this journey
in my return to Hell.

I am truly wasted now . . .

I need all of you
to be such beings . . .
for this one more journey back
to Hell
and through the gauntlet of ravages
so that I may come to life anew,
changed forever,
fighting forever.

And while listening to the birds warbling as dawn crept into
the darkened sky, I also reread your memorials to Max Roach
and Raul Salinas and felt strengthened by your words of your
friendships with Roach and Salinas and their multi faceted lives;
I felt energized by your words on innovation, of friendship, love,
creativity, enduring warrior spirit, suffering, pain, oppression,

of jazz mimicry versus the struggles/obligations to re-create, to liberate. Through your hellish experiences, pain, suffering and utter despair, you continue to persevere and give us life.

My dream of your struggles and your newest compositions for some reason reminded me of Ezra Pound's rendering of the Confucian Odes—a capturing of and perpetuation of trials, tribulations, struggles, joyfulness, humor—words on text without tunes, but words rendered as music recalling lost tunes and melodies, but awaiting renewed voices and harmonies.

My apologies if sharing this dream with you, my brother, is disturbing in any way, but I thought that I should share this vision of you rendering passages from your Cancer Diaries into song— songs of innovation, of gritty honesty, of experimentation, of the experiential, your voice in the "alphabet of omens" that Samoan poet Albert Wendt captures in his concrete poetry called Black Star.

Please let me know what we can do from here. I'm sending some CDs and books, including Laieikawai, Potiki, and Na Wahi Kapu o Maui.

Love,

RICHARD, JEN, KAI, AND MELE

And to the following kokuas for all of their gifts of money, time, friendship, food and beverage, flowers . . .

Thanks to Jayne Cortez for another generous financial gift and informative article on alternative cancer treatments; to Ben Olguin visiting from San Antonio, Texas, who brought donations from himself, the Esperanza Peace and Justice Center and Resistencia bookstore; to Royal Hartigan and Wei-hua Zhang for their cash donation; to my parents, Franklin and Frances, as well. Stephanie Hughley sent me a terrific book about nutrition, *The China Study* by Colin Campbell, . . .

And to my *kokua* pals Mike Surdej, Magdalena Gómez, Stephanie Athey; to the many friends who have brought by flowers, groceries, household supplies and meals, including Paget Walker, Joanne Maffia, Sean Lewis, Jen Shyu, Soomi Kim, David Kastin, Lisa Yun, Ali and Sylvie Shames-Dawson, Jennifer Kidwell; and the juice sent by Parker Pracjek; visits by Tom Buckner, Bobby Zankel, Joe Russoto; the letters, cards, and financial contributions by Dolly Veale and Baraka Sele; delicious lunch cooked by Melanie Dyer and the new CD from her husband and my college buddy; the composer-tenor saxist-scholar/professor Salim Washington; the many bottles of San Pelligrino and Trader Joe's Blu Italy mineral water brought by Robert Adam Meyer, Karen Zhou and Corky Lee, Ashley Byler and Stephen Jackson; the visits and flowers from Marina Celander and her family; the cooking of Gladys Serrano; the outings to Flushing Chinatown and Sunnyside Turkish restaurant with Mike Surdej, Abraham Gomez-Delgado; the terrific books and CDs from Hawaii from Dennis Kawaharada; and the Hamasaki-Dang family.

And to my *kokua* Peggy Choy who for nearly two weeks helped me do household chores, be my secretary, watched movies with me, and gave me vigorous conversations. She anticipated all my needs, struggled with me to stay optimistic, accompanied me, and took copious notes in my meeting with urologist Dr. Aaron Grotas, shared laughter, meals, and ideas for future collaborations.

Finally, I would like to tell you about the publication of my latest book, the anthology *Afro Asia: Revolutionary Political and Cultural Connections between African Americans and Asian Americans* (Duke University Press, 2008).

DIARY 20: ROAD TO THE FUTURE—A LIFE IMPOSSIBLE!

July 19, 2008

August 4, 2008, will mark two years in the war against cancer that I have fought, though it is projected that the colorectal cancer tumor had begun to grow about ten years prior, around 1996.

In these two years, I have gone through four surgeries. The first two, performed August 25, 2006, and March 25, 2008, were to remove the original tumor (which when originally discovered via the first colonoscopy was roughly the size of a golf ball) and the recurrent tumor that had apparently returned to the exact same location less than a year later and less than three months after the first six months of FOLFOX chemotherapy had ended. The third surgery was an emergency outpatient procedure to unblock the ureter to my left kidney with the insertion of a stent. The blockage was found in a routine CT scan performed on July 1, 2008, possibly caused by the six weeks of daily radiation treatment and/or from the accumulation of two surgeries, for which scar tissue and trauma have resulted (the left side of my back, where the left kidney is located, is very closely located to where the tumors have been). The fourth and hopefully final surgery will be July 31, 2008, to remove the ileostomy bag and to reconnect my bowel.

I have gone through three rounds of chemotherapy, utilizing six out of the seven available chemo drugs presently used in Western colorectal cancer treatments (the seventh drug is a duplicate of one of the other six), for a total of forty weeks of bombardment. Not to mention the weeks of postchemo side effects and detoxification trauma.

I have gone through six weeks of daily (thirty days) of radiation combined with daily chemotherapy.

During these past two years, I have suffered many physical losses, yet have gained invaluable and indelible transformation of soul and consciousness, and ironically, even with the physical losses, a new and better physical being.

These have been the physical losses:

1. Constant, though lessened since the original FOLFOX chemo round, peripheral neuropathy: slight and constant pain and numbness to my feet and hands, worsened with cold and contact with metal, glass, and other conductors of cold. Even holding metal keys in my (ungloved) hands worsens this condition. Though recently, holding my saxophone seems not to be a problem.

2. Much slower growth of bodily hair: I shave perhaps once or twice a month now.

3. Inability to ejaculate. This condition may be temporary. The urologist said that within a year's time, it may return, but should it not within that time; then it may never.

4. Left kidney blockage, which requires a new stent and outpatient surgery every three to four months for now. Hopefully, in time, the stents have permanently kept the scar tissue from congealing and no longer be needed, but again, this is uncertain.

5. Thickened scarring on my abdominal surgical incisions of a foot in length from the two surgical procedures that opened the front of my belly for the tumor extraction and colon resectioning: my stomach scar is very tight and restricts the flexibility of my abdomen.

The transformations and gains in my life and body are the following:

1. The journey to eliminate all ego from within me: to accept being flailed at by invective and tirade, no matter how unjustified, and to seek out the grain of truth that might be present;

2. Getting off the treadmill of career and competition and comparison; to no longer desire nor seek acceptance or legitimacy from the establishment;

3. To allow love, integrity, courage, and the pursuit of excellence be the core of my life and relationships;

4. To no longer eat any meals after 5:00 PM; to exercise constantly; to eat foods that are considerably less from animal sources; to drink fresh juices, mineral water, and teas; to eliminate as much as I can from eating processed foods; to shop for foods daily and especially at farmers markets that sell locally grown and harvested foods;

5. To live with less material belongings, to purchase as much secondhand and recycled merchandise as I need or want, to live at the level as much as I can as that of someone of a middle-class standard of living in the third world as part of struggling to live in an ecologically sustainable paradigm;

6. To appreciate and enjoy all my friends as my circle of love, who have all helped to keep me alive and made life worth living for;

7. To do my work without regard to compensation or personal rewards of any kind except the satisfaction of knowing that I am doing my mission on this planet, which is to do the music and political activism that no one can or will do;

8. To live without fear, envy, jealousy, or insecurity;

9. To never again live with any kind of orientation toward the past but to focus my energy entirely upon the future: to bring into being that which needs to be done, even though it may be impossible or no one else may do (for now): to imagine and do the impossible!

On July 31, 2008, I go for surgery to remove the ileostomy bag and to reconnect my bowel. I am expected to stay five to seven days in the hospital and then discharged for home recovery. I am supposed to have a visiting nurse come to my home daily to help me repack the open wound. I am planning to recover in those few weeks before I depart on August 27, 2008, to Madison, Wisconsin, to begin my teaching residency at the University of Wisconsin. I plan to use the fall of 2008 to rebuild my body and to begin life anew on January 1, 2009. I will begin to fulfill my bucket list and to live and do the work of living an impossible life.

(For those who would like to visit me, I'll be at Beth Israel Hospital, Sixteenth Street and First Avenue in Manhattan. Just drop by. Ann Greene and Paget Walker will be asking people to stay and/or visit me at home once I'm discharged to help with chores and errands.)

DIARY 21: A SLOW RECOVERY AND HEALING—
CHALLENGES AND THE UNKNOWN OF A NEW LIFE

December 1, 2008

First, my apologies for not sending out a cancer war diary entry for some time. Several of the Warriors for Fred LISTSERV have inquired about my condition, as they haven't received what was once a weekly to monthly blog from me. A new frontier has begun for me with many uncertainties and unpredictable challenges that I will detail below.

Second, as part of the newness of everything in my life, which I am very hesitant to call "postcancer war," I have been struggling to figure out how to best describe and philosophize about "what's next."

Lastly, I have been focused on trying to get better healthwise and physically, as well as to be better in my attitude and activity in this transitional period.

Let me fill in what has happened.

ILEOSTOMY REVERSAL: GONE, FAREWELL, AND NOT TO BE MISSED!

On July 31, 2008, I returned to Beth Israel Medical Center for my fourth and, hopefully, final in-patient surgery to remove the much-disliked ileostomy bag I had hanging from my upper right abdomen as part of the treatment to allow my cut and shortened bowel tract to heal from two resectionings performed to remove the initial and recurrent colorectal tumors.

I couldn't wait for this day as the bag was a shackle. My life, both waking and sleeping, revolved around it, always anxious that it might leak, overfill, or, worse, completely break or fall off. Every few days, it needed to be changed, and I dreaded the possibility of the stoma (the intestinal extension "nipple" that siphoned my feces externally) spurting while the old bags were being disposed of and new bags were being prepped for attachment. Supplies had to be regularly ordered. I couldn't go swimming in a public pool for either people seeing me with a bag and/or objecting to the "what if" of the bag leaking or breaking off. However, I did manage to go twice to the beach and swim in the ocean briefly without mishap. The day of July 31 was a truly joyful feeling. The four months of having the bag was misery at worst, and constant anxiety at best.

During those past four months, I had to find restaurants with clean and large-enough men's rooms to change the bag after a meal. Again, so many wonderful friends came by, picked me up, and drove to great places to eat in the new foodie mecca of Queens. At least, I could now enjoy food again.

Whenever I did go out, I had to bring the ileostomy supplies with me in case of bag problems or cleaning myself when the bag filled up immediately after eating a meal.

The other constants I had to adjust to were sleeping at night only on my back so the bag wouldn't be punctured or broken. I also changed my eating schedule to not eat after 5:00 PM so as not to have the bag get too filled during the evening and sleeping hours. Ironically, this habit has proven to be a blessing from a curse. I had lost thirty pounds since the surgery to remove the recurrent tumor and install the bag, and that weight has stayed off. Eating at night, especially before sleeping, has been shown to have several negative health effects. The effect of *not* eating after 5:00 PM has kept my intestines clear and clean at night, allowed for better nutrient absorption, diminished weight gain, among other health benefits.

Additionally, it has been a spiritual-philosophic reminder to me: to empathize and know what it means to go to bed hungry at night, as most people on this planet experience. I am constantly reminded of my journey to eliminate ego, accumulation, and the profligate.

Finally, because I had the ileostomy bag during the hot summer months, I did not want to wear pants over the bag due to both the discomfort and the extra anxiety it caused over the possibility of breakage; instead, I wore long flowing, breezy "robes" (the Egyptian galabias or the West African *bubas*), which were both very practical, comforting, and easily hid the bag. But by wearing such clothing, I learned the awful experience of homophobic hatred and violence.

Once walking the streets of my Greenpoint neighborhood, an older Polish woman sneered and ranted at me, "Wear pants! Wear pants!" I was stunned and was at an unusual loss of words to respond. To my defense, a young man in his twenties or early thirties shouted at her, "Don't be an ignorant bitch!" I was being defended against hatred and prejudice by the use of additionally and equally derogatory speech!

A similarly ironic experience happened in Harlem in late August. I was sitting on the brownstone stoop of my friend and fellow musician Dr. Salim Washington's home. Joining us was an elder friend of Salim's who was self-admittedly homophobic. (Earlier in the afternoon, I overheard him describing his dislike of Wynton Marsalis and the cabal of jazz at Lincoln Center as a "bunch of faggots." I confronted him and asked him if he was homophobic, to which he admitted with candor that he was.) We were simply talking about music when a young teenager threw a brick at me (my back was turned to him, so I didn't initially see it). The brick missed me and fortunately didn't hit anyone as it smashed against the brownstone exterior wall. Both Salim and his friend yelled at the kid. Salim's elder friend advanced to confront the youth, and the two got into a shouting and daring match of calling each other faggot. Later, I surmised that my genitalia were exposed in the way I was sitting on the stoop and that the youth took offense to that. I later shared with my friend Sue Bernstein this troubling experience. Sue made a brilliant recommendation: to create a piece possibly titled "Fly Free, O Genitalia! Fly Free!" I loved the idea and made it an assignment for my students this fall where I am teaching at the University of Wisconsin–Madison.

So the bag finally came off. Again I had to be cut open. More scar tissue. Lying on my back a day after surgery in the recovery room, I was shocked to see the hole to which the bag was attached. I was stunned to see how big it was: about 4.5 inches in diameter and just as deep. I could literally stick my hand in it and touch my intestine. Ann Greene was present with me in the hospital when I saw it for the first time, and I called it my "crater." It was a blow to me to see such a large and deep hole. I was worried that it would take a lot longer to heal and seal up than the twenty-seven days I had when I would get on a plane to fly to Madison, Wisconsin, to begin my teaching. When I was discharged and sent home to recover, the visiting nurse assigned to me told me about the Medi-Vas, a machine designed to accelerate wound healing via suction of debris, increasing circulation and aeration. The machine was ordered, but before it arrived, an emergency situation happened.

MYSTERY VIRUS: MY TEMP RISES TO 104 DEGREES

After five days of being home, with the loving care and help of General Ann Greene coming over daily to attend to me, I started to feel very weak and tired, barely able to stay awake much less do anything. When the visiting nurse came and took my vitals, my temperature had climbed to nearly 102 degrees (fever is considered 101.6 degrees). I called Dr. Picon's physician's assistant, Margo LeStrange, who urged me to check myself in at the Beth Israel Medical Center Emergency Room. She said she would facilitate the check-in so I wouldn't have to wait the many hours so typical to emergency room walk-ins.

Ann stayed with me as I went through the emergency room admittance, tests, and scans. Dr. Picon came by and noted that I really didn't look well. Only by using ice packs did we seem to stabilize my body temp. I had entered the hospital early afternoon, and by 1:00 AM I was transferred to a special floor. Ann stayed with me until about 1:30 AM.

I was experimenting there in my treatment, as none of the doctors seemed to have any certain idea of what was causing my temperature rise. And it was still climbing. I knew that a body temperature rise that exceeds 104 could be deadly and that covering one's body in ice would help curb that temperature rise. I kept insisting that the nurse fill trash bags with ice. Some nurses were cooperative while others weren't. At one point, my temp did hit 104, and it was clear to all—doctors, nurses, and specialists—that something terribly wrong was happening to me. Standard antibiotics weren't working. Scans did not indicate any infection with the left ureter stent that was recently put inside me back on July 7. The other possible source of infection was my Medi-port (the subcutaneous port that allows for the drawing of blood and chemo infusion), but scans didn't seem to indicate any infection there either.

So with Ann Greene's help, I got the nurses and aides to fill up multiple layers of garbage bags with ice and covered my whole body with these makeshift icepacks. It helped. My temperature would drop 2 to 3 degrees.

After three to four days in the hospital, my temperature held steady below 100 degrees. Melanie had arrived to stay with me. I asked to be transferred to a VIP room, which I would have to pay for, about $175 per night, to spend the next two nights in luxurious privacy without the noise and constant interruptions from the other patients with whom I had to share a room in the regular recovery suites. Also, the food was much better, as it could be ordered off a menu. Eventually, I was told by Dr. Picon that after all the test results had come in, that no specific cause could be ascribed to this alarming condition. I was discharged home after five days in the hospital.

While in the hospital, a Medi-Vac had been put upon my open wound, and it seemed to work miracles. I could visibly see that the machine was accelerating the wound healing. I asked the visiting nurse service to continue this treatment for the time I had remaining at home before departing to Madison, Wisconsin.

LEAVING FOR THE MIDWEST

Early evening on August 27, 2008, I had to fly to Madison to get set up there for my fall guest teaching position. On the morning of that day, my longtime friend Sarah Dupuy came by to help clean my apartment ceiling fans and do errands. That afternoon, Ann, her sister Lois, Lois' daughter Lilli, and Mark O'Ferrall all arrived to help me clean and prepare my apartment, as I would have subletters stay there for the duration I was going to be away.

We had an early dinner at a nice French restaurant in Long Island City before my departure from LaGuardia Airport.

I had wheelchair service at the airport, which was a big help. I didn't think I could carry my sax and carry-on luggage and walk the distance through security and to the gate. I got on the plane and was in constant discomfort and mild pain from sitting up at a right angle for three hours. When I arrived near midnight in Madison, Peggy Choy met me to help carry my bags to her van and drove me to my new studio apartment.

When I entered the apartment, I noticed the small size, about two hundred square feet, and the cheap construction and obviously worn condition from student tenants. The night was hot and humid, and Peggy turned on the air-conditioning. I spent an hour unpacking and setting up the apartment and then fell right asleep. The next few days were spent getting my faculty ID and other bureaucratic errands. I could barely walk three blocks. The Medi-Vac had helped lessen the size and depth of my open wound, but it was still about half an inch deep and two inches long by an inch wide. I was also in constant pain from the stitches and the wound itself. For the first two weeks, I continued to wear a wound dressing, which I changed and put on daily.

I discovered that Madison has a Trader Joe's where I would get most of my groceries and a great outdoor Farmers' Market on Saturdays that wound around the state capitol, about five blocks from where I lived. The first visit, I had to sit and rest constantly, with Peggy carrying all my bags of produce.

My studio apartment is on the top floor (tenth) with a nice view overlooking Lake Mendota. The place is inhabited mostly by students of the university. Thursday to Saturday nights would be loud partying, but I was high enough from the street that the noise wasn't too bad.

I began teaching my first class on Tuesday, September 2.

TEACHING, MIDWEST ALIENATION, AND THE NEW FRED HO

The time away from New York City has afforded me the chance to get more rest, to use the athletic facilities, to reflect and meditate upon the combination of great physical losses and concomitant philosophical gains from the cancer war, to gain experiences as a visiting professor, to make new friends among some faculty and with all of my students, to recognize that my recovery would be much longer and more gradual than I had ever thought, and to realize that I could never go back or even bounce back to the life I had before. That the concept and word "back" was impossible. We can never return to the past, only move forward.

It became crystal clear to me, as I announced in my first return trip to New York City to perform at the BAMCafé with my band, the Afro Asian Music Ensemble, that "The old Fred Ho died on August 4, 2006. That was my predecessor. I'm the new Fred Ho."

The course I am teaching at the University of Wisconsin–Madison, a Big Ten campus with over forty thousand students, is called Revolutionary Afro Asian Spoken Word and Performance (listed as Asian American Studies 260 in the course catalog). My duties as visiting artist in residence sponsored by the Arts Institute, with co-sponsorship from the Asian American Studies Program, the Department of Afro-American Studies, the School of Music, and the Department of Dance and Drama, is to teach twice a week on Tuesdays and Thursdays.

My Tuesday classes are what I design as theory classes where I mostly present and lecture and the students discuss the materials and ideas I present. Thursdays are practice classes designed to be performance and rehearsal laboratories where they improvise, collaborate, and work on performance techniques.

I disagree with grading, but had to subvert the university requirement for grades by making a deal with the students that I'd give them all A's, but it was their responsibility to keep that grade or plummet together. This was lesson one in accountability and collective collaboration.

Second, my goal was to replace grading with a commitment to the following: excellence, imagination, integrity, and courage.

Third, I want them to be daring revolutionaries, to never regurgitate, revise, rework, redo—i.e., hold on to the past—but to boldly take on the future of creating new work and new processes and social relationships as a precursor to building a new society.

Last, I wanted them to treasure and fixate upon creative innovation as artists and producers. To see education and their lives not as passive consumers in which teachers, the media, or society tell them what to think, consume, and do—but to be active producers in self-learning through collaborative and collective interaction and to make the culture they believe society needs and to create the better world that they envision. I told them, "My job is to kick your ass so that you can eventually kick my ass and make me obsolete." One of my requirements is to have them write their own manifesto: what they believe and what they want.

I really got into teaching and have been very excited about these ten undergrads. I have three men and seven women, four Euro-Americans and the rest third world people (a Kuwaiti, two Asians, two African Americans, one Latina). They self-selected themselves as I required any students interested in my course to audition. The purpose of auditions is not to see what they have done or can presently do, but to assess how open they are and their potential. Naturally a number of students were culled because they didn't want to audition or take a course that focuses upon performance.

There was one grad student who initially begged me via e-mail to accept him, citing a litany of credentials coming from the prestigious New England Conservatory and being a recipient of a financially lucrative D.M.A scholarship from the graduate department of the University of Wisconsin School of Music. But when he got into the mix with the undergrads, I believe he was intimidated by how much more creative and daring they were, and he quickly dropped my course. It was obvious that he couldn't think/create outside of the box or his familiar comfort zone.

As I've come to see the work of these ten wonderful undergrads, I realize that while I may not have the best poet, the best dancer, the best actor of this campus, I have the most imaginative. Their exciting work made me feel that perhaps teaching would be my next calling as I embark day to day upon my new existence. However, as the semester progressed, I have come to realize that I am better suited to teach informally (via my cultural work and via special one on one or small group processes at my home, such as study groups) than via a formal institution such as a college or university. Why? Because I'm a vanguardist! I do my best when working with those who want to learn from and be involved with an explicit "far left-winger" like myself whose methodology is anti mainstream. I also can't stand being around careerists, of which there are many in academia. I also can't go along with the rules and general parenting and coddling and hand holding that are generally expected of teachers with even adult college-age students. I would consider an offer from an institution if the following three non negotiable requirements of mine are met, and the fourth is my preference but not required:

1. I teach what I want to teach. It would be a waste, for example, for me to teach Music 101 as plenty of career-seeking faculty can do this. My unique experiences and expertise would best be utilized in such courses as Revolutionary Lessons of the Black Arts Movement or Opera for a New World, etc.

2. I take no more than fifteen students. For education to truly be interactive, collaborative, and transformative, only in small groups can this be done. Otherwise, it is a lecture or presentation that inculcates mimesis and not debate and struggle.

3. The students must audition, even if the course is primarily theoretical or a symposia. I want to cull out those who are simply looking to fulfill a requirement or who only have an intellectual curiosity instead of a willingness for self-transformation, deepened commitment, and action.

4. (Optional) Pass/fail, no grading. Academia, as in all avenues up the ladder in stratified society, is a process of getting through gatekeepers instead of self-production and independence. The adage of students performing for the test more than the intrinsic value of education and liberation is promoted by the pursuit of grades. Education reflects the economics of a capitalist society: as Ivan Ilyich describes in the metaphor of banking—the accumulation of deposited information for cumulative profit or gain, rather than my criteria of excellence, imagination, integrity, and courage.

The students finished their semester in a major performance by creating individual works, some in collaboration with other students, woven together by myself into a piece I titled as "Future Forward Suite: The Revolution Is Political, Personal, and Cellular!" This was presented on November 22, 2008, to an audience of almost eight hundred. My band, the Afro Asian Music Ensemble, came in a few days before, and we rehearsed with the students.

I was so thrilled and happy for the students, who blossomed and exploded. They all turned corners in their artistry and in their personal development. Some of the highlights: a limited-English-speaking Korean woman student created the first modern Korean folk opera like work, writing the text herself and performing it in a glorious tradition-like folksong style. I have waited an entire lifetime to find someone in the United States of Korean descent who can do this. What a breakthrough for her personally and for creating a groundbreaking advance in form. A mixed-heritage Japanese and Euro-American woman created a magical realist mythic epic poem about a selky-mermaid-like entity. An African American woman sophomore created, from one of assignments to write a tall tale (á la John Henry, Pecos Bill, Paul Bunyan, etc.), what I think will be considered a new American classic, "Brotha Brown," based upon legendary nineteenth-century abolitionist John Brown (see her text at end of this war diary entry). A Jewish American woman student created "Fly Free, O Genitalia!" (title thanks to Sue Bernstein) based on an assignment I gave on this title from the earlier-described incident of my being gay-baited in Harlem this past summer. Her work was critical of the sexual conservatism of Israel seen as a by-product of its colonization of the Palestinians. All of the students' works were exciting, bold, daring, and transgressive.

The process of working together in my class created a special bonding and mutual respect among all of us. To varying degrees, all of our lives have been changed together. Here is what I believe to be the significant breakthroughs:

1. Among themselves, the students were openly critiquing one another's work in order to *not* fall into what they called "stereotyped hip-hop spoken word" styles. Initially I was simply hoping that they would be open to moving beyond the "stereotyped hip-hop" styles and form limitations, but they went further to embrace originality and finding their own individual styles.
2. They all created original new works that combined individual expression with sociopolitical vision and imagination; they did *not* regurgitate, revise, redo, or rework past creations.
3. They demonstrated collective accountability by helping one another, as well as criticized one another to achieve collective improvement.

Their continuing problem remains punctuality, getting work done by due dates, and not having forward vision to think, plan, and prepare ahead of immediate tasks and assignments. In part, I believe this problem is endemic to the atrophy of long-term commitment, responsibility, and vision that has resulted from the domination of cell phones, text messaging, e-mails, all of which enable *procrastination and wait-until-the-last-minute-ism*! That is Fred Ho the Luddite ranting!

The greatest gratification for me has been seeing the development and transformation of these young people and the confidence I feel about them and the lasting friendship we will all have together.

The one other gratification of my long stay in the Midwest (four months has been way too long for me as I'll explain below) is making new friends, especially Dr. Sandy Adell of Afro American studies; Dr. Henry Drewell, an African art history scholar and his wife, Sarah Khan, an alternative medicine and food specialist.

Other than the students and these new friends, I have to say that *I greatly dislike* the Midwest and don't want to return unless for lucrative revenue needed to fund my projects.

Here is what I so dislike about the Midwest:

1. Bad food. The blandness and tastelessness is rooted in the subsequent points.
2. Obvious monoculturalism.
3. Meek and weak third world people. Essentially, there are no physical concentrations or communities of Asians, blacks, Latinos, etc., in a Midwest city such as Madison, Wisconsin.
4. Arrogant whites!

For the first time in thirty years, I felt like a minority again, and not simply due to the numerical relationship. The only time I don't feel like a minority is actually in my class with the ten students! I am constantly personally affronted in liberal Obama-landslide Madison. From rudeness by whites to actual discrimination. I have seen the effects of being called a chink by undergrads who were upset by the grade they received from a fellow forty-something male Asian American studies professor—how that experience and his failing to beat the hell out of those racists has psychologically grated at him, causing him to lose tenure, fail to publish the book he was writing, and continue to wallow in the lowest faculty rungs. I see arrogant white undergrads talking back to me, trying to get in the last word when I am a fifty-one-year-old visiting guest faculty of this university.

For the first time ever in my life, I was racially profiled for being an Asian American man in an Asian restaurant by the white female manager. She yelled "Where are you going?" as I tried to join my dinner party upstairs (for which we had a table reserved) and I calmly told her that I have a reservation and was simply joining my dinner party. She became so defensive, citing that she couldn't be a racist because she has an Asian boyfriend, and besides, so many of "those people" come off the street into her restaurant. I questioned her as to who she meant by "those people." And sticking her foot deeper into her mouth, she answered, "Those people who dress like you, you know, with a hoody sweatshirt, sweat pants, and sneakers" (I had just come from the gym). I pointed out to her that she had no sign requiring dress attire and that this twenty-something white man sitting behind me was dressed in a baseball cap and T-shirt but was never spoken to in the manner that she did to me. To her credit, she comped the dinner.

I later learned that a former waiter, who is an Asian American student I met on this campus, has filed a complaint against the restaurant for stealing tips and withholding wages. I and others have encouraged him to vigorously pursue justice.

I can't wait to return home to multicultural New York City where the racism I fight is more macro and institutional and not daily personal indignities.

The one good thing I think Madison in particular has that can be complimented is a very good health care industry. The doctors and overall experiences I have had have been very good.

SOME OTHER NON-MIDWEST HIGHLIGHTS

I returned twice to New York this fall—in mid-October to perform at the BAMCafé, the NYU Slave Routes conference cultural event curated by Jayne Cortez and a book signing event at Magdalena Gomez and Jim Lescault's home in Springfield, Massachusetts, for the *Afro Asia* book and the 2009 Sheroes calendar. As soon as I landed at LaGuardia,

Joseph Yoon picked me up and drove me to Flushing Chinatown for a great feast. The Asian food in the Midwest really is awful.

I came back mid-November for the world premiere of my concerto for baritone sax and orchestra, "When the Real Dragons Fly!" at Carnegie Hall/Zankel Hall. That was a wonderful experience with a great performance by the American Composers Orchestra. The *New York Times* said the "[b]luesy harmonies and thunderous brass riffs recalled the work of composers like Charles Mingus and Archie Shepp" and that I "looked healthy and played with abundant energy. In his brawny solos he testified and roared with unbridled passion, and the orchestra served as an exuberant congregation."

THE FUTURE

I have my colonoscopy on December 8, 2008. That will be a very important test. Should the tumor return, then my condition is certainly metastatic, and I may have to accept a terminal condition. Should I be clear, then I can have some relief until the next colonoscopy three years from now. If I can stay clear ten years, then the probability of my being a certifiable cancer survivor will be very good.

You will all hear from me shortly and in brief after December 8.

All my love!

FRED

BROTHA' BROWN (A Tall Tale) by Dominique Nicole Chestand

Old John Brown
Never wore locked chains
On his wrists
But the hills of Virginia
Screamed cries
For the noose he wore
Round his neck

Brown fought the heat of the South
With such passion
That the fire in his eyes
Would melt chains
Covered in plantation mud
And weld them into guns of liberation
Some say
That when
A member of the Brown family
Was born
The melanin
Would wear off their skin
As midwives
Cleaned the flow
Of their mother's womb

But the name Brown
Stained Old John's blood
So deeply
The images of his darker counterparts
Ran through the veins
Of his retinas
And cried freedom
So loud
It shattered the stars
On Confederate flags

DIARY 22: THE WAR CONTINUES—CANCER AGAIN ATTACKS FRED HO

December 15, 2008

My annual colonoscopy was performed December 8, 2008, while I was teaching at the University of Wisconsin–Madison by Dr. Chip Foley. He informed me on Wednesday, December 10, that a mass was found but was not certain whether it was benign or malignant and sent a piece of it for biopsy.

Dr. Foley called me Monday, December 15, 2008, first thing in the morning, and told me that the biopsy results confirmed that cancer cells were present.

I will meet with my oncologist Dr. Peter Kozuch here in New York City on Friday, December 19, 2008.

Meanwhile, I have been very busy assembling a super big band of my favorite musicians over the past twenty-five years to record on December 17, 2008. Should I live or die, I wanted to perform at least one more time with these musicians and decided the best way was to assemble *all* of them and hence do a big band recording project. It will be the first release on my new record label, which will be a special subsidiary of new music philanthropist Tom Buckner's record label, Mutable Music. In preparation for my possible expiration on this planet, I hope to issue a spate of recordings and publications. My lack of physical fortitude will probably limit my ability to mount large-scale operatic works as I have been doing since the late 1980s.

I go and visit my family after meeting with Dr. Kozuch.

I ask that all of you refrain from contacting me until after January 2, 2009, so I might have some peace and contemplative space to figure out the next phase of the war.

All love,

FRED HO

DIARY 23: HOPE REDUX

January 21, 2009

To all my dear friends, I want to thank you for your love and friendship in respecting my wishes to have space and time during the last weeks of 2008 to spend with my family and to allow me to focus on the myriad of medical tests and appointments required by the finding of cancer cells in my colonoscopy of December 8, 2008.

I know many of you have expressed to Ann T. Greene and directly and indirectly to me your continuing love, support, and concern for this latest news.

In the past four weeks, I have had many tests, and finally, today, I have some final conclusions, for which I will get a second opinion in the next two to three weeks from colorectal surgery specialists at Memorial Sloan-Kettering Cancer Institute. Here is what we know for sure:

1. I do not have a metastatic condition; the suspicion of pelvic bone cancer was not supported. *That is terrific news!*
2. The cancer in my colon is most likely not a recurrence, but a new occurrence, which from all examinations, including biopsy and endorectal ultrasound scan, to be "superficial," about 1 cm with almost no depth, and as far as can seen discerned via these tests, without penetration. Its actual depth will only be ascertained once surgery is performed. *This is also terrific news!*

It means that, for now, the recommendation by the Beth Israel doctors is that I have a "trans-anal excision of rectal mass" procedure, a minor surgery that will not require cutting me open again (!) but excising the cancer growth via my anus. I could quite possibly return home that day after the procedure and recover in a couple of days at home.

I will be scheduling a second-opinion consultation with Memorial Sloan-Kettering within the next two to three weeks. Should there not be a differing opinion to the above, then I am scheduled for this surgical procedure on Thursday, February 12, 2009, at Beth Israel.

For the first time in this brutal war, there is a real medical basis for hope in a cure for me. However, I am cautioned by the Beth Israel doctors that once I am opened up and the cancer is closely examined, should the tumor be of more depth or extent that initially believed, that the treatment may move to a more draconic procedure of permanent colon extraction/removal and the installation of a colostomy bag for the rest of my life.

Obviously, I would greatly prefer this does not happen, that cancer does not return, then, at last, after more than two years of a brutal war, a hope for curing me will be very real.

Below is a commentary I originally gave verbally to my students at the University of Wisconsin–Madison, for my one-time, first-time-ever course I created, Revolutionary Afro Asian Spoken Word and Performance (Asian American Studies 260), as part of their overall group evaluation. The students asked that I write it and send it to them for closer reflection.

FINAL PRESENTATION TO THE STUDENTS OF FRED HO'S REVOLUTIONARY AFRO ASIAN SPOKEN WORD AND PERFORMANCE (Asian American Studies 260, University of Wisconsin–Madison, December 11, 2008)

After hearing you read your Manifestos as the last assignment for the class, I have the following collective comments:

Change is never easy, always difficult and hard, always requiring sacrifice.

Yes, change begins with the individual, indeed at the cellular level, and if it is to be real and genuine, insistently at the cellular and must extend far beyond the individual into the social and engage the entire universe. That's why real change is and must be total and fundamental.

Limited, partial, cosmetic change (i.e., reforms), whether monumental or momentary, risks being reversed or perverted unless the fundamental—i.e., the majority of the conditions to measure that change—are maintained, perpetuated and in constant revolutionary development.

While I realize you are young in life, the dominant perspective regarding change in your manifestos still focuses on "I" the individual. There is some inclusion of "we," almost none on "the world" (both human and other life forms). The second you understand you, the particular, as a participant in the universal, and no longer place primacy upon the "I," but rather upon "we" and "the world," will action and imagination become united.

Honesty is laudable but insufficient. To be honest that your shit smells doesn't make it perfumed or aromatic. It still smells bad. Beyond honest criticism and analysis, real knowledge is both activist and collaborative. Activism is practice or action and is the sole criterion and test of truth. Consciously united with theory, it is called "praxis." Can you prove it by making it real, even if simply at a beginning level. Collaborative because to acquire universal knowledge requires sharing and anti selfish and anti egocentric investigation, testing and experimentation. That is why a journal, taking notes, being punctual (respecting your colleagues and participating every second) is crucial. Otherwise, everything is simply relative, disconnected, and a collection of diverse opinions, but no primary direction or course of coordinated, united action.

Professionalism is a form of technology—actually, a mode of organization that seeks optimizing diversity through differentiation. It is not the Namby Pambyism of letting all opinions have equal weight and mired in liberal lowest common denominator choices and courses of actions. Rather, the technology of professionalism is optimizing human excellence, integrity, imagination and courage. Making money is an-almost side thought or by-product of this optimization.

Technology isn't just machines. The greatest technology is human creative labor. Our ideas, social organization and spirit or will. In the tall tale of John Henry, the individual man beats the machine, but the machine comes to rule the day. What we need is a lot of John Henrys.

Here's my differentiation of the ten of you: One is ready to join the professional ranks, without any doubt as to skill, talent and professionalism. What is lacking for this person is the ability to give leadership: when chaos, confusion and crisis abounds, to step forward, and as asserted by Muhammad Ahmed, to take command. Not to make everyone a follower, but to weld the ensemble so that all excel and advance far beyond the sum of individual talents and efforts.

Another person has much of the professionalism, perhaps the talent, tries to exercise leadership, but is perhaps too focused on personal relationships without sufficient inter connection to the world.

The rest of you have potential and promise, but lack the basic professionalism to yet enter the world as serious contenders. Some also have the excessive self-involvement of "I" and fear sacrifice and continual, relentless struggle, especially as it comes to facing the challenges of the planet that dwarf the challenges of previous generations, e.g., global warming, lack of clean drinking water, the death of the coral reefs, etc. The mere accumulation of good deeds or simply not offending anyone or someone doesn't challenge the status quo. It *is* the status quo.

You have all kicked my ass. I couldn't write this if you hadn't. But I apologize that the institutional boundaries of my being an employee at this educational industry didn't allow me to kick your ass harder, as I would have surely done in the world. But given what the rules of engagement are in this training or practice environment, with most safety protocols in place, we've challenged each other fairly well. But if this were my home, where I prefer to teach, and have done so for thirty-plus years, we might scream and yell at each other, and the next minute kiss, hug and make love.

That is the struggle over contradictions. It never is easy. It is how change is made. It always is how real knowledge happens.

I had an interesting discussion with Prof. Michael Thornton yesterday who taught me the distinction between the discourse and conception of "challenge" versus "struggle." Challenge implies choice. Struggle, there is no choice. Fighting cancer, for example, is not a challenge, but a struggle (indeed, a war) as there is no choice. The only choice other than to fight or struggle, is to die. That isn't a choice. We fought for Ethnic Studies and for liberation overall because we had no choice. Otherwise we'd remain corpses, the lobotomized coerced labor for our oppressors and exploiters.

DIARY 24: TROUBLE ON MY MIND

January 12 to March 13, 2009
Difficulties and Determination

This cancer war diary entry has been the most difficult to write, and it may be the most difficult for some of you to read. I caution anyone that the details and admissions I make herein may be hard to accept.

I returned from teaching in the Midwest on December 12, 2008, filled with satisfaction for the work I had done while an artist-in-residence at the University of Wisconsin–Madison. I was also very happy and excited to be returning home to New York City. The day after I returned, I plunged into massive rehearsals with the Green Monster big band, a new large ensemble I had assembled, to do a new recording of my extended big band compositions, a project I am calling *the celestial green monster*. As I explained to the twenty musicians at the beginning of our first rehearsal, I am uncertain whether I'll live or die from this cancer war, but I wanted to be together with my favorite musicians and record again with them. Since there are a number of them, a big band project seemed a good way to do this.

Because I believe so strongly in the necessity of rehearsal, we worked for three days straight and knocked out the project in less than seven hours in the recording studio, with a lunch break of fabulous food catered by my dear friend Paget Walker and assisted by Christina Hilo.

During the holidays, I visited my family outside Washington DC, while taking the Amtrak Acela regularly to New York for a myriad of doctors' visits and tests.

In early January, after a renal exam, my urologist, Dr. Sovrin Shah, informed me that my left kidney had pretty much ceased to function (still alive but only working at 11 percent of functioning, with my right kidney doing 89 percent of the work). The left kidney had been poisoned by the accumulated treatments I have had, especially chemo and radiation. This was not good news, but I can still live and function with only one (the right) kidney—another physical loss to the growing list of losses I am encountering. Dr. Shah suggested I have the stent in the left kidney ureter be removed to prevent possible future infection when I have the surgery for the new tumor that was found at the December 8, 2008, colonoscopy.

But on January 12, 2009, a new complication began that has plagued me and confounded my medical team. A terrible exhaustion and fatigue has immobilized me. Since that time, I have had little energy, barely able to function at the most basic level, often sleeping from twelve to sixteen hours a day. I went into a meeting with Dr. Kozuch, my oncologist, and Dr. Picon, my surgeon, at Beth Israel Medical Center, and I was feeling so badly, my blood pressure astronomically high (160/110), that Dr. Kozuch felt I should be sent to the emergency room. EMS arrived and wheeled me there, and after half a day of testing, nothing was found and I was sent home. The mystery of this severe and enormous tiredness I feel continues as a mystery, one that I feel needs to be solved, as it took me on a spiral of downward depression, which I will convey shortly.

During this time, the good news I received from my Beth Israel medical team was that this new tumor was not a recurrence of the two previous tumors, but what they call a "new primary," and from all the tests, small in size, located far from the anastomosis (the resectioning location of the past tumor removal surgeries), very near the edge of my colon and anus. This gave me a big boost of hope, shared with all of you in the last entry.

The Beth Israel doctors encouraged me to get a second opinion. Since I have been living on federal Social Security disability for two years, I now became automatically enrolled in Medicare (the federal government program that pays 80 percent of most medical costs of eligible U.S. citizens over age sixty-five or like myself, unable to work at all, and surviving on the $673 a month of disability payments from the U.S. government). The remaining 20 percent is to be covered by New York State Medicaid. With Medicare, I now became eligible to see most doctors and hospitals throughout the United States, including the much-vaunted Memorial Sloan-Kettering Cancer Center (MSK) whose slogan is "The best cancer care anywhere."

Before an appointment with any doctor at MSK can be made, they require the entirety of your medical records be sent to them. This was relatively easy, as I had been earnest in keeping my records and notes during the more than two years of this war. I was given an appointment to meet with colorectal surgeon Dr. Jose Guillem for late January 2009.

Initially, I believed the constant debilitating fatigue I faced was from a flu virus of some kind. But after two weeks, I was not getting better. I had very little energy. In the first year of this cancer war, I could expect and look forward to a few weeks of "good" with vigor and energy, which I zealously took advantage of by practicing my sax, composing, reading, writing, exercising, swimming, and enjoying myself. What were once weeks now in early 2009 had turned into days. Those few good days I had I tried to exercise, swim, practice my sax, do a little bit of organizing, and producing. It seemed finding those good days became fewer and interminably farther apart.

I consulted all my doctors. For the most part, my medical numbers seem very good. All the tests seemed to indicate no metastasis, no diabetes danger, generally very good blood pressure numbers (though prone to occasional high swings, but for the most part, pretty good), blood work seemed to indicate no deficiencies, etc. My primary care physician, Dr. Chao Chen, told me that he thought I was just in a bad loop from the massive hammering that I have had over the past two and a half years, without a break. All doctors felt that I have done remarkably well given all that I have faced.

But I still continue to feel awful, tired, and the very life force within me being drained. I felt I was going to die, despite the medical facts to the contrary (i.e., no indication of infection, metastasis, small new tumor, etc.).

For the first time in this brutal cancer war, I was trapped in a vortex of depression, feeling I could not win, that I was getting worse, unable to do anything (from brushing my teeth much less creating music, even unable to type this to all of you). I began to feel suicidal—that giving up and dying would be preferable to living at a minimal existence. I had a hard time thinking I could talk to anyone about these thoughts of despair and hopelessness.

I went to MSK to meet with Dr. Guillem with my sister Florence. MSK is a very impressive facility—the minute you enter, a friendly doorman opens the door and greets you—a Maya Lin-esque designed lobby with stone and waterfall landscapes most floors, waiting areas are vast, comfortable, and replete with nice beverages and snacks. The staff is courteous and very punctual. Dr. Guillem was very prepared and our discussion was very detailed and meticulous. Because I was now eligible for MSK, I decided to transfer my entire treatment and care there. Dr. Guillem confirmed the opinion of the Beth Israel team that I would need a "transanal excision of a rectal mass" whereby the tumor would be excised through my anus, foregoing the need for major surgery like what I had previously. He was also hopeful that the tumor would be superficial at best or, at worst, not deep in its penetration of my bowel lining. He told me the procedure would be a day or two, and we scheduled it for February 19, 2009. I also requested that the left stent be removed, per the opinion of Dr. Shah from Beth Israel urology. He agreed and his assistant got a Dr. Touijer from MSK urology to do this. Dr. Guillem also connected my oncology care to Dr. Zsofia Stadler, whom I met and had detailed discussion of my situation a week later.

I was excited, hopeful, and eager that this surgery seemed to be easy and would not take a long recovery period. Or so I thought.

With sadness, I informed Drs. Kozuch, Picon, and Shah that I was now going to be treated by MSK and thanked them and the entire Beth Israel staff for their professionalism, kindness, and friendship.

During the course of the next month, I would regret transferring at least my urology care to MSK. Since I have vowed not to devote much of my precious little energy to negative situations, suffice it to say, that after enormous efforts by myself and my friends, that the urology physicians and staff of MSK were very disappointing, and after weeks of effort to find satisfaction, including calling upon MSK Patient Representative and Social Work staff, I decided that I no longer had any confidence in these folks and left. I will continue my cancer care with MSK doctors Guillem and Stadler, but my urology care would return to Dr. Shah at Beth Israel.

Just to share the extremity of the contrast in responsiveness, after weeks of trying to get phone calls returned, questions answered, and appointments made, I called Dr. Shah's office on Tuesday, March 10, at 9:15 AM and his assistant, the kind and cheerful Loisita, scheduled me to come in that day for an 11:00 AM appointment. Dr. Shah promptly met with me, ordered tests, and set an appointment for a cystoscopy for March 17 at 8:15 AM. Whew, what a relief and what a satisfying experience instead of the hassles and what I angrily told the MSK patient rep was the obstructionism I encountered from MSK urology.

The surgery went smoothly on February 19, but new problems manifested immediately.

That day, I was supposed to have two procedures: the excision of the new tumor and what I thought would be the permanent removal of the left kidney stent. Before and after the procedure I never once met or talked with the urology surgeon, who, just as I was about to have the procedure, I learned was not Dr. Touijer, the urologist I had come to believe would supervise my urological care, but Dr. Herr. Instead of a permanent stent removal, I learned just before going under anesthesia that I would have a stent replacement. Postsurgery, I was informed by Ann T. Greene who companioned me during the day and into the evening, that it was reported to her that pus was found around the stent that was replaced. Could the stent have caused an infection that might explain all of the heavy fatigue from which I was suffering for the past five weeks? No one from urology could answer our questions.

Dr. Guillem informed Ann that the surgery was successful, that the tumor was removed with margins (additional tissue surrounding the tumor to make such wandering cancer cells would be extirpated).

Because no adult patient beds could be found for me immediately postsurgery, I was sent to the pediatric ward. The one good thing was that that ward was very quiet. A testament to the superior consideration of MSK, the nurses at least closed my door after they took their tests and administered my medications. I was resting until 3:00 AM Friday morning February 20, 2009, when massive incontinence began. I was rushing to the toilet every fifteen minutes with uncontrollable diarrhea. This would continue for hours.

Later the next morning I got to meet my roommate, a teenager who had his leg amputated from cancer in his knee. I apologized to him for the noise I made during the early hours of the morning with my frequent rushes to the toilet, for which I had no control and had several times shat on the floor. I was also lying in my feces. When the night shift nurses got off, they didn't bother having the morning shift clean and remake my bed.

I hadn't eaten for forty-eight hours and was famished. MSK gives you a menu, and I have to admit, their food service was very good in quality. I ate breakfast and later an early lunch before Paget Walker came by to accompany me in my discharge. By midmorning, the diarrhea had stopped, and I was now suffering from constipation! I was also in considerable pain, which made walking and sitting in a car seat very difficult.

While waiting for the discharge protocols, I got to talking with the teenager with whom I shared the room. In all my experiences in cancer wards at three hospitals (first, Long Island Jewish; second, with Beth Israel; and now MSK), I have come to recognize that perhaps an even greater danger than the cancer itself is the loneliness, desperation, and despair of the patients. This teenager needed to really talk to someone, and I provided him that someone. He just talked and talked. I realized that everyone has a story, their own cancer war, and they are yearning to tell it, for someone to listen, to understand, and maybe have compassion. Though he had lost his parents, his uncle and aunt, who had children of their own, and as I learned, worked several jobs, were supporting his treatment at the very expensive MSK, paying out of pocket as he had no insurance. I remarked to him that he was fortunate that his uncle and aunt cared enough to be shelling out tens of thousands of dollars for his care. Part of everyone's cancer war is having someone to talk to. To share your worries, fears, questions, frustrations, and affirmation your humanity.

He was venting to me that the chemo he was taking made drinking anything hard for him because whatever he drank, including water, tasted awful. I told him he had to keep hydrated since our bodies are 70 percent water (as is our planet) and suggested that since he liked and could eat fruits, to find his hydration that way. I gave him my four key fronts in the strategy to fighting cancer, which I wrote about in the first year of the cancer war in this diary: hydration, nutrition, oxygenation, and love. He liked the way I, for the most part, rhymed these points.

When all of the protocols were completed, I had to say good-bye to him. I was very eager to get home, sleep in my own bed, and in my mind, proceed aggressively toward recovery as I had planned to fly to the Bay Area on March 1, 2009, to perform.

It soon became apparent to me how wrong and mistaken I was in my expectations for a speedy full recovery.

At home, I was suffering from alternating constipation and incontinence. I was also in tremendous constant pain. I couldn't lay on my back due to the pain of my anus touching any surface. I had to lie on my sides. For two weeks, I could only lay in bed or on my sofa-couch, but *not* sleep. For the next twelve nights, to about 5:30 AM, I was constantly going to the toilet. It wasn't diarrhea, but the frustration of feeling an impending bowel movement, but with considerable difficulty being able to evacuate, and when finally able to do so, releasing small, rabbitlike pellets. I would think that my bowel movement was done, return to lie down, and then feel it coming on again. This cycle would repeat, in a maddening and painful and frustrating repetition throughout the night. Only by midafternoon the next day, from complete exhaustion, would I get three hours of rest, but never full REM sleep. This was hell again.

Sitting in a chair for more than a few minutes was unbearable. On top of the pain, with the sleep deprivation, I could barely expend any mental energy to talk to people, much less even reply to e-mails. I couldn't figure out anymore how to do daily life tasks such as check my mail, make food, answer, and talk on the phone.

Since January, no longer did I have good weeks or even days, but if I was lucky, simply a few good hours a day, and many days, not even that, maybe a few minutes to answer a couple of e-mails, speak on the phone in short sentences, struggle to pay my bills, or eat something.

I was *not* getting better. I felt like I was getting worse. I finally came to embrace the two soul-shattering notions: how it could be better to have one's entire colon removed and live with a colostomy bag and be rid of the pain and constant incontinence and, I must admit, the desire to commit suicide. To not live a life or existence filled with pain and inability to be productive, much less to even handle one's own life responsibilities. I was laying in my own feces at home, my bed and sofa coach covered in newspapers and padding.

I decided that my hopes and excitement for resuming my activities as a performer could not happen, so I called Tom Buckner, Jayne Cortez, and many others with whom I had made plans to do performances and speaking engagements, that all had to be indefinitely postponed. Everyone was sympathetic, understanding, and actually agreeable. They knew better and accepted more than I could, that I really need to focus upon recovery and getting better. But what was destroying me from within was the intensifying doubt that I may not get better, that the end of my life would be next.

Two weeks after the surgery, in the few good moments I had, I was fighting MSK Urology to simply get either the surgeon on the phone or a face to face meeting to answer my concerns about the pus found on the removed stent and the question of the stent being a cause of infection and my terrible malaise. This ordeal was the epitome of frustration and the cause of anger boiling inside of me, of the high-falutin' establishment institution and hire lings more concerned with publishing their fancy-ass research papers and high-profile cases than returning a patient's phone call or listening to their concerns and questions. Whatever energy I had for recovery and healing was being consumed by a volatile and destructive mix of suicidal desires and the desire to unleash myself as a terrorist self-exploding maelstrom against the MSK urology department. I was the perfect recruit for a suicidal bombing against them.

Two weeks following my surgery, I met with Dr. Guillem. Aib Gomez-Delgado was my companion for the entire MSK visit. What transpired would dramatically help me turn the corner and give me clarity and thus, a better focus and direction than anger and frustration. Dr. Guillem had postsurgery explained to Ann Greene, who explained this to me, but given I was foggy from anesthesia, did not hear, much less comprehend the following:

> Because of the massive scar tissue inside of me, there was not enough skin tissue in my bowel lining to sew me back up again. The pain and alternating constipation and incontinence was due to this condition.

At last, now I understood! I asked him how long the recovery would take. He said, "Very long." I then asked, "How long is 'very long'?" He said, "I don't know." I appreciated the candor. I now knew that the hopes and expectations I had of a minor surgery and what I thought would be a quick and easy recovery were not going to be. I now could easily postpone everything I was hoping to do for the first half of 2009. I now knew I needed to rest, recover, and focus on my treatment. I now knew I had to call upon my circle of love (all of you) for help and support during these very long months of pain and difficulties.

For the first time in a month, two nights ago I was able to sleep for eight hours. Today, because I was up all night evacuating my bowels, I can sit by my computer and type this cancer war diary entry.

Dr. Guillem clarified to me that though the recovery would be long and difficult, that I would recover, heal, and get better. Even though the mystery of my intense and obdurate fatigue remains, I am not preoccupied with struggling with MSK Urology and have gone back to Dr. Shah.

But I am different now from this awareness and realization: I know with confidence that I will get better. I am determined to get better. And getting better, I now understand, means putting aside my plans, travels, and the things I was wanting to do, but focus entirely upon rest, recovery, happiness, and more rest. I now know that this is what I need and *want* to do. Once the body heals, I can exercise again and rebuild my physical being. I can practice again. I can compose again. I can proceed to tick off my bucket list, etc.

Before this latest onslaught began, I was able to complete three important things, which I hope all of you can check out and promote:

I wrote two speeches, "Trouble on My Mind: New Challenges for Afro Asian Ascension" (which would have been presented at two conferences this spring) and "Future Forward: A Vision for Revolution" (which would have been presented at the Labor/Community Strategy Center event in Los Angeles as a discussion about a vision of socialism that should be, in my view, both matriarchal and Luddite). As always, your critical feedback is always welcome.

And my newest book is being published by the University of Minnesota Press, *Wicked Theory, Naked Practice: The Fred Ho Reader* by Fred Ho, edited by Diane Fujino, foreword by Robin D.G. Kelley, afterword by Bill V. Mullen.

Here is the back cover of the book:

Wicked Theory, Naked Practice is both the remarkable autobiography of writer/saxophonist/activist Fred Ho, as well as an impressive treatise on black musicians and jazz that touches on every possible topic from Cal Massey to current Asian American musicians and the sixties movement. (Yuri Kochiyama)

Fred Ho writes as a revolutionary Asian American artist–activist for whom his music and his politics are inseparable parts of his identity. All his life, he has been seeking to navigate between the Scylla of a Marxist universalism that ignores oppressed nationalities and the Charybdis of a cultural particularism that ignores the urgency of political action. His search has led him to advocate a struggle for matriarchal socialism. This is urgent reading for all serious activists. (Immanuel Wallerstein, Yale University)

Fred Ho's *Wicked Theory, Naked Practice* is an important work, with critical understanding of the most advanced arts/cultural, political social wave of the last part of the twentieth century and the actuality of a new reality and promise for the twenty-first century, his own errors notwithstanding. (Amiri Baraka)

For more than three decades, Fred Ho has been a radical artist and activist. As a composer and saxophonist, he is famed for creating music that fuses Asian and African traditions. The influence of the black power and black arts movements inspired him to become one of the leading radical Asian American activist-artists. *Wicked Theory, Naked Practice* is a groundbreaking collection of Ho's writings, speeches, and interviews.

Fred Ho is a composer, musician, scholar, and activist. He was the first Asian American to receive the Duke Ellington Distinguished Artist Lifetime Achievement Award.

Diane C. Fujino is chairperson and associate professor of Asian American studies at the University of California, Santa Barbara.

Robin D. G. Kelley is professor of American studies and ethnicity at the University of Southern California.

Bill V. Mullen is professor of English and director of American studies at Purdue University.

I know I will get better; I know that to get better the difficulties will be painful and hard, but I am determined to confront them because I know I will get better.

DIARY 25: DO THE IMPOSSIBLE TONIGHT AND SLEEP . . .

May 25, 2009
FORWARD HO! Getting Better Day by Day

After about six weeks from the last surgery I had on February 19–20, 2009, my body turned a major corner and it began an accelerated healing. During those six weeks, as detailed in the last entry, I had gone to hell again, faced the devil, and almost surrendered this war. Though the tumor was a T1 (small, only penetrating the bowel lining halfway), because of the accumulated treatments of multiple surgeries and chemo/radiation bombardment, I had a massive amount of scar tissue that prevented my surgeon, Dr. Guillem, from sewing me back up and had to heal naturally.

With a dozen sleepless nights, tremendous pain, constant bowel movements (as many as thirty times a day, as frequently as every fifteen minutes) and extreme tenesmus (explanation below), hammered exhaustion, depression, and frustration, I felt that anything would be better than what I was experiencing, which included coming to accept having a permanent colostomy bag if it came to that (a leap of acceptance given how I hated the temporary ileostomy bag I wore for four months last year), and worse, having thoughts of suicide, believing death would be better than the agony.

But I remember exactly when I turned the corner for the better. My *kokua* Peggy Choy had flown to New York from Madison to stay with me and help with chores. That Saturday morning, after only a few hours of sleep, I woke up feeling energized and really wanted to help Peggy with the cleaning of my apartment. So I went out as the stores were opening to find a good wet mop to clean the floors. Only a few days before, it was painful to even walk, much less sit erect in a chair to type on the computer or even read e-mails of any length. I came back and Peggy was not pleased that I had gone out while she was still sleeping to perform this errand. I complied with her insistence that I lay down and rest. After cleaning the apartment and having a light breakfast we made plans to connect with my friend Joe Russotto in the East Village for an early dinner (I have been eating before 6:00 PM to try to minimize the number of bowel movements through the night in order not to constantly interrupt sleep and run to the toilet all night).

After Access-A-Ride dropped Peggy and me off, we met Joe, and I was feeling excited and eager to finally get out of the limited three blocks of my neighborhood that I could barely walk for the past six weeks, that I asked if we could walk around and sight see. We found a great Italian restaurant and enjoyed a delicious meal. I was very anxious that my bowel movements would be erupting in havoc, but since I had scheduled our Access-A-Ride pick up with about an hour to spare, and the restaurant was packed and needed us to vacate our table after finishing our meal, we cautiously walked around the area. While I felt full, I didn't feel like I was going to burst, as had been the case after I ate during this awful time.

Access-A-Ride came, and we returned to my apartment in Brooklyn. I undressed and immediately went to the toilet. At first, it seemed it would be painful and difficult again to do my bowel movement. But for the first time since the surgery, I was evacuating in steady, vigorous cycles. Because of the multiple colorectal surgeries, my bowel tract has been reduced in length by sixteen inches, so the movement in the shortened tract now moved in smaller and quicker waves instead of what is for normal people, a continuous single pushing wave.

That evening, sitting on my toilet, for once I was able to completely clear out my colon, and felt for the first time totally relieved! What a joy! I felt an inner confidence that I could finally go to sleep that night without constant interruption and could really get a full, complete, good night's REM sleep. And I did.

MISSION: IMPOSSIBLE!

The open wound was healing and mending. I was careful and cautious to not get too excited. I had been down that road before, thinking I was on the mend, raising my hopes and expectations, only to be slammed back down with symptoms of a returning cancer tumor. But this time, after postponing all my travel and public engagements for the entirety of 2009, and dedicating myself to the focus of healing, recovery, and improvement, I have been uplifted to feel and know that I am on a very good path now. Daily I improve, not just physically but also in my soul and spirit. I now have accepted what it means to be off the treadmill of pursuing career, accumulating income, caring about what the music and art business wants or deems worthy and important; and I have embraced *love*, of always spending time (a lot of it) with friends, family, and people who want a just, equitable, and better society. I am also completely accepting of my *mission* for the remainder of my time of this planet: to do the music/art and politics that no one can or will do! I have fully committed to what Sun Ra insisted: that since everything has been done and nothing has changed, what is needed is the impossible. I continue to struggle to eliminate ego, to focus on the future and not the past, to work on doing the impossible.

I was supposed to be dead a year ago. My oncologist, Dr. Zsofia Stadler, admits that my case is very unique and unusual, that I've tried all the chemo drugs that Western medical science has invented for my stage of colorectal cancer, and it has become apparent that none of them have worked; that, as she admitted, you couldn't find a hundred cases like mine throughout the world to even conduct a reasonable clinic trial; and that I will not be out of a danger for some time, perhaps for my entire life. That I continue to be here, to do what I do, to make the personal transformations and to achieve the internal transcendence that I have, that is doing the impossible. I realize that the impossible is a constant work in progress, a process, and a journey, never to be fully measured, quantified, or completed.

MEET THE NEW FRED HO

As I get older in age, more hammered by the cancer war, and suffered the many physical losses, the gains I have made in my consciousness, spirit, and imagination and vision have made me *better*. I am convinced of this. That's why I now always introduce myself as "the New Fred Ho." I couldn't have come thru this war without having killed the old Fred Ho, to have fully committed to repelling all the toxicities of capitalist existence (the treadmill), to accept the new possibilities no matter how impossible. I continue to fight on.

On the sociopolitical-cultural level, I am even more dedicated, outspoken and ferocious, but the old Fred Ho, shaking with rage and anger at the system and its accomplices, is gone, and the new Fred Ho is now saturated with a tremendous love for all who contribute by their deeds towards advancing the struggle for liberation.

The old Fred Ho denounced Ludditism. The new Fred Ho IS a Luddite (again, not antitechnology, but opposed to technology that is harmful to people and to the planet).

The old Fred Ho would have ego and, conceit, and exhibit arrogance at indignities, affronts, injustices (both socially and particularly targeted to himself), explode in anger and fulminations at inadequacies and improprieties. The new Fred Ho is highly selective, only chooses to be involved with the vanguard of integrity and excellence, regardless of stature and mainstream legitimation.

The old Fred Ho was a polemicist (see *Wicked Theory, Naked Practice: A Fred Ho Reader* to get a sampling of this!). The new Fred Ho is a philosopher and seeker.

The old Fred Ho was unsatisfied, wanted to achieve more, accomplish more, believing that somehow, through sheer dint of his determination and tenacity, that the mainstream would accord him something. The new Fred Ho doesn't care for any of this and is only focused on his mission.

I believe that one of the carcinogenic factors of the treadmill was the pursuit of success, often to the detriment of health and happiness (internal peace, without the toxicity of anger as the predominant emotion—anger at injustice and at compromise and complicity with the status quo). The new Fred Ho now understands the distinction between success as "getting what one wants" and happiness ("wanting what one gets"). Competition, envy, anger, covetousness (both overt and covert), ego—the new Fred Ho is on a journey to eliminate all of these toxins.

The only two public engagements that I kept for spring 2009 were two book signings/performances for the publication of *Wicked Theory, Naked Practice: A Fred Ho Reader.* The first, held on May 7, took place to a packed attendance at the Asian American Writers Workshop in

Koreatown, Manhattan. The second, organized by the great Magdalena Gómez, was at the Holyoke, Massachusetts, Barnes and Noble. Both events had terrific turnouts and sold out of books. A book celebration and cultural event also happened, organized by Peggy Choy, at the Asian American Studies national conference in April in Hawaii, for which it was not possible for me to attend as I was unable to even sit in a chair for more than a few minutes, preventing me from making a long flight to the Hawaiian nation. Reports are that it went well and books were sold. I have made it a point to sign each book with a unique epigram, to never repeat myself, just as when I improvise on my saxophone, to not repeat myself.

For two events that I had postponed, a conference on American studies at the University of Texas at Austin, and the aforementioned Asian American Studies conference in Hawaii, I had drafted a short speech titled "Trouble on My Mind: New Challenges for Afro Asian Ascension."

Because I couldn't be there in person to deliver this talk, two friends who are professors of Asian American studies read my paper at these respective conferences. The feedback I got from the two friends who are professors of Asian American studies was that some if not most of the attendees (who are professors or aspirant professors of Asian American Studies) objected to my essay. The Texas conferees felt I was too binary in my thinking by posing the positions as authentic versus sellout. While at Hawaii, the feedback was that my essay was not nuanced enough.

For a few days I personally wrestled with this feedback. I realized that I had drafted this piece early this year, prior to the last surgery, and had intended to revise and work on it some more, but the severity of the postsurgical recovery was far worse than I had expected and precluded me from even sitting in a chair for any length of time to write at the computer. I am fighting to eliminate ego so I was soul-searching to ascertain if my being troubled by this feedback was personal vanity and ego. But after conversations with some of my *kokua*, especially one who is seeking to rise further in the ranks of academia, I began to recognize that the accusations of binary thinking and lack of nuance have more to do with the aversion of academics to real struggle (and by extension, accountability and responsibility) about *the stand* one (must) take in the gutting of commitment towards Asian American liberation (and by extension, the liberation of all oppressed peoples for which queer, ethnic and working class studies were conceived and constructed to primarily support).

I believe that the accusations of my being binary is a recrimination of me for taking a stand, and the charge of "not being nuanced" is that I actually carry out and fight for what I stand for. As always, yours or anyone's direct feedback and commentary to my ideas are always welcome, either by a direct phone call or in-person conversation, or via e-mail (though as a Luddite, I refrain from spending more than five minutes in e-mail discourse).

As the weather gets warmer and the sun rises earlier, I am day by day feeling better about everything. I awake each day after a good night's sleep, never to go to sleep with anger or anxiety, and to avoid eating after the sun goes down. I eat smaller meals, mostly raw food (fruits, vegetables, fresh-squeezed juices, unprocessed nuts, raw fish), though I still remain an omnivore and occasionally eat pork, some chicken and turkey, low-temperature-cooked foods. I swim at least twice a week, do light exercises, and practice the saxophone at least five days a week. I have begun to write music again, just completing a big band arrangement of Jimi Hendrix's "Fire" and working on an extended arrangement of Hendrix's "Purple Haze," which I am reinterpreting. Instead of the common understanding of "Purple Haze" as the stupor and intoxication of drugs, I reinterpret the song to mean the stupor and intoxication of false consciousness, or of the condition of "being in the matrix." I'm collaborating with Randy Wolff for this big band arrangement.

One of my immediate projects is to finish this collection of cancer war diary entries for my book. My intention is to make this an instruction manual and philosophical tract for fighting the twin, interconnected, interrelated plagues of cancer and capitalism (which, as my woodsman friend Jay Crotchett has pointed out to me, are the same inextricable processes of accelerative malignant growth). As I get better, I will embark upon more projects and activities to realize my mission. But for 2009, the main goal is to get better. Because of the frequency of tumor growth for me, I will now have biannual colonoscopies. I have one scheduled for August 5,

2009, and a later one will occur either in December or January of 2010. I am determined to have these tests come out clear, which will be the first time for the past three years. If both are clear, I will proceed into 2010 with a myriad of activity, as the new Fred Ho, free of carcinogenic-generating inducements, and immersed in peace, satisfaction, happiness, fun, mostly raw food, Ludditism, and love.

Daily I get better, in terms of physical and psychological improvement. Besides the persistent peripheral neuropathy (pain in my extremities, viz., fingers, and feet), which diminishes with warmer weather, I continue to have a condition Dr. Stadler has described to me as tenesmus, the feeling of having to move my bowels all the time (brought on by the greatly shortened length of my bowel tract after the multiple surgical resections). I try to evacuate my bowels as thoroughly as I can each time I sit on the toilet, but it never seems that it is thoroughly cleared, so I have this persistent feeling of needing to crap again.

Beginning this summer, one day a week, I plan to work on a farm and in exchange for my free labor, get my food sources directly from what is grown and prepared there, which will include hand-threshed wheat/flour, pork from pigs I slaughter, vegetables, etc. I also plan to swim at least twice a week in the ocean and begin to plan the launching my own Internet television station featuring music, the arts, and progressive-radical sociopolitical ideas.

On May 27, 2009, I was honored by the Brooklyn Borough President's Office as a notable Asian American resident of Brooklyn during this year's Asian Pacific Heritage Month celebration. I remember about thirty years ago when then-president Jimmy Carter made the official recognition of the month of May for Asian Pacific Americans, after such ad hoc, unofficial celebrations had been organized for years prior by our communities, including the Asian Pacific American heritage celebration in New York City and the Asian American Awareness month that I had conceived and initially organized while a student activist during the mid-1970s. The May 27 event was surreal and bizarre with Brooklyn Borough President Marty Markowitz constantly sticking his foot in his mouth, conflating all Asians to be Chinese, noxiously promoting the model minority myth that Asian Americans have made it in America, and for his obvious lack of any basic knowledge of Asian American history. He also was slovenly sucking up to the consulate person from the People's Republic of China, furthering the misimpression that we Asian Americans are either all recent immigrants, foreigners, and again, all Chinese.

The eye-candy hostess, a local TV newscaster of Asian descent, never left the green room, fixated and Tweeting on her BlackBerry, so she misattributed the obvious South Asian youth dance group as Chinese folk dancers. As usual, Asian Americans get token attention, and when there is even that scant attention, clumsily stereotyped and presented with so many sloppy inaccuracies. Such errors are like the thinking that Africa is a country.

HERE'S FARMER FRED

I have recently begun working once a month for a week on an organic farm in the Delaware County of the Catskills to grow my own food. It is very hard and grueling labor, and given that my strength and stamina is not what it was, I can only work about four hours a day. But breathing the fresh air, getting vitamin D from the sun, working my muscles, and enjoying the simple but delicious organic vegetables and fruits is a great joy and learning experience for me. I had several epiphanies while working on the farm. I realize how defrauded we all are by capitalist factory farming and food processing that we are denied the taste of real food, and how good that food can really taste, as well as denied the benefits of greater nutritional density from such food and the way it is grown and gotten to our kitchen tables. I also realize that organic farming without any petrochemical fertilizers or pesticides requires a lot more labor, which is why mass production farming is cheaper, but not better. The greater labor required by organic farming would mean more employment, especially without the hazards of chemical toxicity to either the laborer or to the consumer. Finally, the reduction of consumerism generated by organic farming: less carbon burned by transportation, less packaging, to even fewer kitchenware as the pure taste of the food requires less involved preparation, and consequently less stuff in the kitchen.

For our meals, we ate straight from the ground. A pasta sauce was simply olive oil and fresh tomatoes stewed on the stove with no salt and pepper, no garlic, no onions, no cheese. And it tasted delicious. Nearby is Arcadian farms, run by a Belgian immigrant man named Laurent. I got some fantastic lamb *merguez* sausage freshly butchered, chorizo pork sausage, lamb ribs, and center leg cut. I met the pigs, ducks, chickens, cows, and rabbits he raises.

Country farm living isn't for the squeamish or neatniks. As my friend Jordan Colon pointed out, there is no separation between indoors and outdoors. We go in and out of the farmhouse with mud and dirt. The house interior is very simple and rough, a place originally built in 1827 (yes, almost two centuries old), probably not cleaned in years. It doesn't have to be that way, but the twelve to fourteen hours of work per day in the fields doesn't leave much time or energy to keep a house tidy and cleaned. The water from the faucet is great fresh spring water. A stream runs through the farmland with a nearby waterfall. On the way there is a patch of fresh thyme. By the time we lay down to sleep, we all were exhausted.

I was especially worn out, being the oldest person there by almost ten years, and having gone through the cancer war. The sun beat heavily on me, and I had to take a break during midday when the sun was hottest. I sweated profusely. I was covered in mud and dirt. Blisters broke out on my left hand. I mostly did weeding, dragging the hoe through rocky but mineral-rich soil. I was often on my hands and knees planting saplings of forty to fifty different varieties of tomato plants, four different kinds of basil, kale, a bunch of different kinds of lettuce, cabbage, asparagus, spring onions, scallions, leeks, chives. The farm also has watermelons, cantaloupes, honeydew, strawberries, squash and zucchini, rhubarb, and other vegetables I probably don't know about.

Jordan is the owner of Eat Records restaurant in Greenpoint, one of the best restaurants in New York City because all of the foods is local and organic, mostly all of it from the farm. He has limited refrigeration and only an electric, not gas, stove. So his operation is very small and limited in scale, but not in quality or taste. The profound nature of his space and equipment limitations requires his cooking, particularly the food itself, to be the best and healthiest. You can Google search the restaurant and read the reviews. The tables and chairs in the place were made by his older brother, a gifted carpenter. The restaurant shares the space with a used record vendor, so it has a bohemian, but not pretentious faux-hipster, feel. It is one of the great assets of my Greenpoint neighborhood.

A program he and other restaurants and farmers have created, for which I am now participant, is CSA (community-supported/service agriculture), c.f., www.straightoutoftheground.com.

People can place a weekly order and pay $30 and receive a bushel of fresh fruits and vegetables from the farm. They have to go to Eat Records or other NYC sites to pick up their boxes. People can also special order smaller quantities or specific items, such as a quart of tomatoes, instead of the mixed box. If you want to join, please contact Eat Records at 718-389-8083.

The only thing that doesn't appeal to about the area of the upper Catskills, and rural life in general, is the small-town mentality and pettiness of the social interactions. There are a growing number of city transplants, but it hasn't gotten as bad as say Woodstock, which is simply a replication of yuppie-infested Park Slope!

The rest of 2009 for me is to recover and get better, work on the farm, finish the cancer war diaries, and pass the two colonoscopies. I am for the first time very hopeful, truly looking forward to 2010 when the new Fred Ho engages the impossible!

As always, I'd like to recognize and thank my loving friends who assisted me during this phase of the ordeal: Paget Walker for constantly coming by to look in on me, transporting me to doctors appointments and grocery shopping; Abraham Gomez-Delgado for taking me to doctor visits and my emotional meeting with a social worker at Memorial Sloan-Kettering where I admitted to my feelings of suicide; Peggy Choy for visiting and doing whatever chore need to be done; her daughter Maya for coming over and cleaning my bathroom; Lisa Yun and Ricardo Laremont for donating some money and treating me to a magnificent Malaysian lunch in Elmhurst; Ann T. Greene for everything she does to help me and keep the Warriors for Fred organized; Gladys Serrano and Tom Buckner for visiting and hanging out. And to my old roommate from my days living in Park Slope, actress Cheryl Lynn Bruce and her husband, the visual artist Kerry Marshall, for making contact again and their generous cash donation.

DIARY 25: REMISSION!

October 6, 2009

Here was the good news from this past August's colonosopy, which was shared in an e-mail blast to my Warriors for Fred:

> From what Dr. Guillem could observe, I am clear. Great news! But, he said that the bowel prep (i.e., the clearing of my colon via expurgated fluid intake) wasn't total so that some of my colon lining was covered, and he couldn't see everything. He recommends another colonoscopy in six months, around February 2010. But there was no major observed problem, such as a tumor protrusion. If there is another tumor or small polyp, it is hasn't grown to be extended and could be found and excised in six months.

The news is incredible. That was the first colonoscopy I've cleared in the past three years, without finding either polyps or the dreaded tumors. Through the summer and early fall 2009 I have had several CT scans, scheduled about two months apart, now stretched out to three month spreads, all of which have indicated "unremarkable" (a blessed condition, i.e., nothing, no problems, no alarms, no red flags, no warnings—nothing!). This is now called the period of *remission*: findings of no evidence of cancer anywhere.

This has made for great joy and excitement for me, and I'm sure, for all of you. As many who have seen or spoken to me these summer months can attest, I'm much stronger, more vigorous, very positive, and enthused about moving forward into the future, committed to nothing "re" ("re"turning, "re"newing, etc.), but wanting everything to be new, free of baggage from the past, moving decisively into greater challenges (which include spending lots of time having fun, being with all of you, snorkeling, constructing precursory socialist forms, learning how to be Luddite, living off the treadmill, etc.).

I've been exercising regularly, both strength training, cardiovascular work outs from swimming, but mostly from spending whatever time I can find to work on Tovey Halleck and Madlyn Warren's organic farm in the Delaware county in the northern Catskills, growing more of my own food, finding new sociopolitical-philosophical creativity for solving the problems of ecology and economics and personal health and freedom.

This has been a major change and development for me, a back-to-basic Mao"ism": I sent myself to the countryside to do manual organic farm labor! While I'm not in need of ideological remoulding (Mao and the Great Proletarian Cultural Revolution's stated intention) as I've always respected manual rural labor, and don't regard it as punitive, I do believe that such a path is necessary for social and personal emancipation. When we respect the earth, how our food and basic sustenance is derived, and actually do work that concretizes that connection of earth-human/personal health-food production, then we emancipate ourselves from the capitalist construction of passive consumer/corporate producer. We begin the path to actually becoming independent producers, which provides the basis for more of us to voluntarily, freely, enter into associations/relations as independent producers, which will become the emerging basis of an entire socioeconomic relationship that eliminates the nexus of money, domination, exploitation, and oppression.

So I try to send myself to the countryside as often as I can. There, I work on the farm, practice my sax, swim in the pond—rarely is there a need for cash or technology (I do admit to checking my e-mails several times a day at the one computer there). I also donate a lot of extra stuff I have had in my NYC apartment and in storage to the farm and its satellite in the neighboring town of Andes at which an artist colony-farm is being developed. Central to my new life is eating *real food, mostly raw, mostly plants and mostly from my own labor*. I have extended the Michael Pollan credo (c.f., *The Omnivore's Dilemma*). (Lately, I've been greatly disappointed by Pollan's celebrity status that seems to have increased a syncophancy to the mainstream and fear/anxiety over being "too controversial" as Pollan has declared his support for Whole Foods CEO John Mackey's attack upon single-payer health insurance. Pollan believes backing Whole Foods is more important than the politics of promoting and making the U.S. health care system universal and a right, instead of allowing the ongoing privileging of the insurance industry's obscene lust for monstrous profits.)

I've added a socialist extension to Pollan: Food from one's own labor, and not from factory farms and a whole system of exploitation of both human labor (workers) and the earth.

I'm now never too busy to work on the farm, grow and prepare my own food, have fun on my own or with my friends, or to take on the challenges of my focus ("to do the politics and art that no one else can or will do"). These are Fred's five: *farm work, food, fun, friends, and focus!*

Since I feel confident about the remission (yes, a "re" word, and so is, ironically, revolution!), I have started up new creative, professional projects, including releasing my Green Monster Big Band CD, *Celestial Green Monster*, writing new arrangements for that configuration for a forthcoming second CD, starting on videos, graphic novels, an Internet jazz TV station, etc.

I have also politically embarked upon developing precursory socialist forms in preparation for the meltdown/collapse of capitalism. In a nutshell, if planet Earth is a spaceship, whether the spaceship will survive (meaning for humans, as quite possibly, the extinction of the human species doesn't necessitate such for other species, indeed, might be a restoration of ecological processes distorted and harmed by human dominance), I want to build shuttlecraft(s) for all of us (the warriors who are on this LISTSERV and others). Perhaps we can eventually create a new home that we won't make toxic.

I hope all of you can come to the big band premiere concert January 23, 2010, at 9:00 PM at the Brooklyn Academy of Music BAMCafé for our CD release party and concert.

As I get more professionally active again, my events page on my website, www.bigredmediainc.com, will announce those activities.

If you are in the Greenpoint neighborhood of Brooklyn, have a meal at EAT, 124 Meserole Street corner of Leonard and enjoy the produce from the farm, or check out the CSA (community-supported agriculture) program at www.straightoutoftheground.com.

The thirty-one cancer war diary entries that have been sent to the Warriors for Fred LISTSERV will be compiled and published as a book, *Diary of a Radical Cancer Warrior: Fighting Cancer and Capitalism on the Cellular Level*. And this entry, number 31, is the conclusion.

All love,

FRED

(A PREMATURE) **AFTERWORD**

From May to August 5, 2009, all of my tests, including a colonoscopy, have indicated no evidence of cancer, which means that I am in remission. These results have delighted me and my circle of love (*kokua*). I continue to be a part-time organic farmer, though beginning to research natural farming advocated by microbiologist Masanobu Fukuoka, which is a step further than organic farming in asserting virtually no human impact upon the relationship between society and the natural world. I continue to perform and create exploring new forms and modes of dissemination, and I have inserted myself more formally into the revolutionary socialist anti–imperialist-internationalist movement, all as part of my mission "to do the work no one can or will do, but what must and needs to be done." I am committed to remain off the treadmill and have taken a food vow to Michael Pollan's edict of eating "real food, mostly from plants," and I've added "mostly raw and to consume less overall." Plus I've added my own socialist directive: to eat food I can mostly grow.

The future is always uncertain, but I face it as a new Fred Ho who is fortunate and happy to be alive, healthy, filled with love, and forever fighting for a society based upon conscience, free love, and which has absolutely no impact upon the natural world. The primacy of the planet and people must prevail over the putrefaction of profit (i.e., capitalism).

The New Fred Ho is now here, born August 5, 2006.

THE NEW FRED HO, SEPTEMBER 1, 2009

Part Two:
The War Continues—
Rejecting the Allopathic for the Naturopathic

DIARY 26: THE WAR RETURNS, THE NEW FRED HO TAKES A NEW DIRECTION

October 10, 2010

After so many years of this cancer war, I have truly come to know the enemy. About three to four months ago, at the start of the summer, I felt that the cancer had returned. My bowel movements were painful, difficult and frequent, and of course, blood was regularly appearing in the stool. The sigmoidoscopy and colonoscopy only verified what I already knew (and dreaded) from an internal awareness I have developed after constant war with the enemy.

On September 22, 2010, Dr. Guillem, my colorectal surgeon, did a flexible sigmoidoscopy exam of me because of my reporting to him of constant blood in my stool for the past three to four months. Both from what he observed and from a biopsy, he found cancer. Later, a colonoscopy performed by Dr. Bratcher confirmed the presence of a 2 cm cancer mass at the same location as the last tumor I had, found December 2008 and surgically removed via a transanal excision procedure in February 2009.

Cancer has returned. It has returned four times in four years, with the longest period of remission from March 2009 to mid-2010, almost a year and half of being clear of cancer.

A CT scan was done immediately following Dr. Guillem's finding and the CT scan was "unremarkable." Constant blood tests also have consistently indicated my excellent health and low CEA (carcinogenic embryonic antigen) numbers.

Dr. Guillem's proposed plan of treatment is to entirely remove my rectum, believing that another transanal excision of this tumor would not be effective, with the consequence of my having a permanent colostomy bag.

My oncologist, Dr. Stadler, believes that while there might be some chemo options, as well as perhaps very pinpointed localized radiation, that the risks are very high for further kidney damage (I now only have one functioning kidney, my right side, after radiation and/or a combination of chemo poisoning created hydronephrosis of my left kidney making it nonfunctional in 2008) and very possible worsening of my peripheral neuropathy (pain and lack of dexterity to my fingers and toes) leading to my ability to no longer play the saxophone, which would be a psychological and spiritual death for me as making music and playing the horn is who I am.

I had a follow-up meeting with Dr. Guillem on October 8, 2010. The appointment was set for twelve noon, but we did not actually meet with Dr. Guillem until about 5:00 PM, a five-hour wait. Clearly he was behind that day, and I was not upset, but sympathetic with his long and grueling day. I presented with him with possible other options, including another transanal excision as well as taking three to six months on my new self-treatment of raw food (which I will explain more below) and monitoring me with more frequent colonoscopies to see if my new self-treatment is effective.

During the last cancer war against tumor number 3 (the second primary tumor), I came to peace about accepting a colostomy bag should that be the only and necessary course. Many people, and I think especially men, hate the idea of a colostomy bag, perhaps regarding it as a diminution of their manhood. I overcame that psychological anxiety and dread over a year ago after the extreme pain during the recovery from the last surgery.

Dr. Guillem believed that no more tests were necessary, after I and Dr. Bratcher, the gastroenterologist who performed the colonoscopy, were asking for the need to perform an ultrasound scan to find out the depth and spread of the tumor. Dr. Guillem did not comment upon my suggestion that I continue on my raw diet and have another colonoscopy in a few months to see if progress can be made via this course.

I knew Dr. Guillem was set in the course he wanted me to take, and I do not blame him or believe he was so adamant from the long day and delays he was experiencing that day. He didn't seem to believe that even having the colonoscopy was of real use to affecting his opinions about the next course of treatment, which is to perform surgery to completely remove my rectum.

We got my sister Florence on the phone to ask Dr. Guillem some questions. She asked what he thought the curative chances would be with the proposed rectum-removal surgery. What I heard from Dr.

Guillem at that moment made me turn the corner to the decision I have now made. He said that he did not know and could not opine one.

Since Dr. Guillem's sigmoidoscopy two weeks ago, I became determined to engage myself in a completely raw food diet after speaking to Joseph Chammas on the phone, the first person I could actually directly interrogate who had stage 4 (metastatic) colon cancer (which included emerging cancer growth on his liver). (Stage 4 is the condition in which cancer has spread beyond one area and which makes tumor removal surgically inoperable). Chammas had gone through the worst chemo-hell with the superdrug Avastin and also had radiation treatment. In sum, he had gone through everything that mainstream (allopathic) medicine prescribes and according to him, not only did not improve his condition, but it also worsened his quality of life.

He had decided to reject the allopathic treatments, took a chance with the Hippocrates Institute in Florida and embarked upon a self-treatment strategy of "starving cancer" by a 100 percent raw food diet that included zero sugars, including fruits, as well as high-oxygenating chlorophyll saturation, along with other methodologies. He is now one year cancer free. While it remains uncertain for how long he can remain cancer free, the fact that I could verify his experience and interrogate him directly was decisive for my new direction.

Two weeks ago I started to go all raw. Now many of you have read and heard from me that I have been a strong advocate of raw food diet. But I must admit, I have compromised and lapsed in my own theory and espousals. As I got to feel better during this past year and a half, I deviated frequently, though still striving to eat a larger portion of my food from raw sources. Last summer, I took Chairman Mao's prescription and sent my self to work in the countryside at Tovey Halleck's farm in the northern Catskills, eating food straight from the ground, full of nutritional density. And I was getting better, with remarkable recovery. But I still compromised. I was weak and taken off course, contradicting my own theory of "mostly raw," frequently consuming cooked foods at my home and in outings to comforting, favorite restaurants.

During the first cancer war in 2006–2007, I consumed large amounts of fruit juices: noni juice, fresh-squeezed orange juice, pomegranate juice, carrot juice, etc. During this time, nagging me at the back of my mind, doubts had emerged, about whether by consuming so much sugar (albeit from natural foods) that perhaps I was actually feeding the cancer instead of starving it. The literature I was then studying strongly advocated the healing properties of antioxidants and these "super" juices (noni, mangosteen, pomegranate as three particularly promoted ones). While I had soon come to reject these curative methods as I could find no verifiable evidence of such, I, nonetheless, still subscribed to their value as a good source of vitamin C and antioxidants, which they are. But they are also high in sugar content.

After my conversation with Joseph Chammas, I decided to commit myself to go 100 percent raw without any sugar sources such as fruit. I found now the decisive imperative that now governs my focus and direction for however long I have to live on this planet: *no compromise.*

In the two weeks' time since I began this, I have found remarkable results and serious improvements to my health. These are as follows:

1. With my increased exercise (swimming and isometrics), significant weight loss and increase of lean muscle.
2. While I have been taking blood pressure-lowering medication as my blood pressure has risen to once dangerously high levels, it has steadily been declining with the raw diet, though given the losses (see below) I have had from the massive hammering of chemo, radiation, and the loss of my left kidney, my blood pressure has always remained problematically higher than it should be, but not dangerously high.
3. My energy level and mental focus and clarity have been dramatically increased.
4. And most importantly, I no longer have tenesmus (the feeling of constantly needing to go to the toilet, but unable to evacuate), and my bowel movements are the best they have ever been during this past four years of the cancer war! I evacuate easily, there is no blood, and most significantly, there is no discomfort between bowel movements.
5. I am now feeling the best I have felt since 1990, which long precedes having cancer!

I have told all this to my doctors. To their credit, no one has scoffed or tried to debunk or dissuade my new raw-ism. And I cannot expect them to think outside of their allopathic professional training and experience.

I respect all of my allopathic doctors; none have tried to dissuade me from my new direction. They all warn me of the risks, which I continue to be well conscious of, that a single cancer cell could migrate into my lymphatic or circulatory system and produce distant metastasis, and should that happen, it might very well make my condition inoperable and completely incurable and most likely result in death for me.

But the most important change in these past two weeks has been my decision to reject the allopathic (mainstream medical establishment) treatment of surgery, chemo, and radiation (cut, poison, and burn).

Here is where I am at now:

In summarizing and assessing the past four years of the cancer war, it is apparent, and admitted by all of the allopathic doctors, that the allopathic treatments have not been curative as a whole. That for all three bouts of chemotherapy, it can be admitted that this massive hellish hammering was "ineffective" (Dr. Stadler). That the radiation I received, while it may certainly have reduced tumor number 2 (recurrence of the first tumor), it came with a tremendously awful price: the hydronephrosis or rendering of my left kidney to become nonfunctioning. Surgery also did not prevent either recurrence I have had. It may have bought me a little more time and some months of wellness where I could have a vigorous life and amount of activity, but it, too, was not a curative solution.

For the past four years, the mission has been to defeat cancer. That mission has not met with success. I was a very good soldier. I followed all of the orders and commands of the mainstream medical community, now clearly too problematic results (see the list of losses below). Now I will no longer take commands, orders, or opinions from anyone but myself. I am now assuming full command of the mission. I will have either sigmoidoscopies and/or colonoscopies beyond the insurance company-medical establishment mandated playbook of acceptable (read: insurance coverable) frequency.

While I continue to "turn pain into power" and live with gusto, clearly the losses have been tremendous, though I have turned these physical losses into philosophical gains, but the fact remains that none of the physical losses will ever be recovered. These losses are as follows:

Loss of the function in my left kidney.

Tortuosity of left side blood vessels and constant pulsations in my left ear.

At times acute peripheral neuropathy, loss of dexterity in my fingers (e.g., buttoning a shirt, clamping necklace, threading a needle, lack of ability to do finer finger tasks), as well as numbness and pain in my toes and fingers when in contact with coldness (metals, glass, cold weather).

Left-side intention tremors (a Parkinson's-like condition where my hands shake and I am unable to have muscular control on my left side).

Loss of libido, inability to ejaculate, erectile dysfunction.

High blood pressure, at one point dangerously alarming with a systolic number of 170 and a diastolic number of 120 (normal is 120/80).

Loss of taste. Most food simply tastes bland and boring to me.

For three weeks now I have committed to an all-raw food diet, excluding all sugar-makers including fruits and certain sugar-making vegetables such as beets and carrots. I will ingest a high chlorophyll diet of dark greens through both eating and juicing. The hardest part of this new path is the temptation and seduction, to which we are constantly subjected by the ubiquity of restaurants and food shops and malls, advertising, etc. And our own psychological weaknesses for our once-favorite comfort foods and nostalgia for industrialized food.

There have been marvelous changes and results already from this new path.

Peripheral neuropathy has considerably lessened.

I have lost a lot of weight and am trim, lean, strong, filled with energy and stamina.

I used to suffer from constant mucous and congestion and have very little of that now.

My bowel movements are no longer problematic as they have been throughout my so-called recovery in which I endured tenesmus— explosive and constantly painful and repeated bowel movements when I can evacuate—and now, no more blood in my stool. I believe that these problematic bowel movements made for this recurrence in which my feces would coagulate in my rectum-anus and created a putrid condition that made the tumor toxic.

And most importantly, I feel the best I've ever felt in twenty years! I am truly the New Fred Ho, not just in theory or proclamation but also in physical fact.

I have decided to forego the rectal removal surgery. I am devising my own treatment from this point forward.

Here is my new direction, which is a logical extension of becoming the New Fred Ho. This is also my *no compromise manifesto*:

1. I will now lead my treatment, completely devised by myself. I continue to keep an open mind, listen to opinions and advice, do my own research and investigation, accept or reject what I decide.
2. I will live with a maximum quality of life, being at peace with my decisions and now finally knowing, using myself as the ultimate guinea pig or laboratory, whether the nonallopathic all-raw path will be decisive or whether the radical surgery will be the key to victory. As suggested by some to do both (have the rectum removal surgery, live with a colostomy bag, *and* continue the raw diet), I reject this as a compromise, as I will never truly know what was decisive and effective.
3. Absolutely no compromise on anything. I am completely at peace, and have been so for a while now, with death. I have a two-year plan for what I want to accomplish should my death come quickly, but during that time, I want to live and fight on my own terms. It is this

simple: I will either live cancer-free fighting the way I chose to fight, or I will die.

4. I have made a significant personal revolution, one that has taken on my skepticism (about raw food), that has rid myself of any vanity or dread (e.g., the colostomy bag and radical rectal extrication surgery), and has given me peace, clarity, focus and iron determination to fight to the very end without doubt, compromise, or fear. I have made myself the weapon and rely now upon my body, mind, and spirit as the instrument to my future, whether I live longer or die sooner.

5. I have embraced the extremism that Malcolm X described about what is revolution ("Revolution is extremism"): I will go to the extreme limits and starve the cancer to death. Simply, I contend that revolutions have failed not so much for the superior might of the enemy, but from the weaknesses and compromises of the revolutionaries.

The previous announcement that was issued via the Warriors for Fred LISTSERV proceeded from the presumption of the allopathic treatment path. That will not occur. I will monitor the tumor growth or diminishment via monthly sigmoidoscopies, ultrasound scans, and by whatever evaluation methods exist. In three months, I will assess this path, this experiment, I have chosen. The allopathic path is still an option *only after* I try my own strategy, and I am convinced it failed.

I have always appreciated and accepted the offerings so many of my friends, family and Warriors for Fred comrades have put forward. The greatest gift has always been your love, support, faith, friendship, and belief in me. Some have been generous financially which will go toward the premiums for a new supplementary insurance I have engaged. Others can donate raw flax seeds, raw brazil nuts, raw almonds, organic greens, etc. Others can offer their visits, conversations, exchange of ideas, prayers, chants, *kokua* support, and creativity.

Here are some things that have truly excited me about my raw extreme revolution:

1. The Raw Extreme Revolution has inspired a new creativity within me. I am discovering new ways to make food without gadgets, plastic and electromagnetic radiation.

2. I have been inspired to truly forego all capitalistic snares and entanglements. Health and wellness should not be monetarily profitable. Period. In going raw, I have spent very little money, getting my organic greens from Tovey Halleck's farm in exchange for my manual labor and free saxophone lessons. I aver making raw food mirror industrial food values by being hip, trendy, chic, and more expensive. The Whole Foods–whole-lot-of-profit syndrome needs to be destroyed. I am critical of many of the alternative treatment centers and proponents/healers (I can't say they are doctors because a number of them have no medical degrees) as they seem extremely implicated in capitalistic profiteering, charging $3600 for two session consultations, or $5,000 to $11,000 for luxury treatment spa-like retreats, etc.

3. Raw means real and self-reliant and self-sufficient. The amount of "stuff" is easily reduced, thereby allowing us to get off the accumulation superhighway that has been posed and positioned as the only path (the main street or road). I will return to the farm. I am now invested in a local organic vegetarian restaurant in my neighborhood (www.eatgreenpoint.com), which shares a lot of my own extremism! I now mostly make my food at home, very simply, with minimal financial cost, and it is delicious and life-changing.

Finally, we have organized a Raw Fight Club to take on ending asthma, diabetes, cancer, and many other ailments, diseases, and weaknesses that plague us individually and our society, all part of our ongoing prefigurative efforts toward constructing new social relations free from the cash nexus, emancipation from capitalism, determined to creatively construct something that is impossible, new, and better. We meet at 5:30 PM every Saturday at my place. Here are our six rules of Raw Fight Club:

1. No compromise.
2. If you compromise, you will be kicked out of Raw Fight Club.
3. Everyone must fight. No exceptions. If you're new, you must fight first.

4. Anyone can join Raw Fight Club. Anyone can leave Raw Fight Club at any time.
5. You must talk about Raw Fight Club.
6. You must fight to win.

Come by and visit and see the new Fred Ho. No compromise, hard as combat steel, more than ever ready to make the revolution!

All love,

FRED HO

DIARY 27: LETTER FROM BEN BARSON

It has been over two months since I have been able to sit down and chronicle this latest stage in the cancer war with its many complications and challenges, which have demanded rapid changes from me in my struggle.

The next few diary entries include correspondences (from a young friend, Ben Barson, who heard about my fourth tumor and the "unknown" chances of my overcoming cancer and the anxiety around my near-certain death and an e-mail I sent to Memorial Sloan-Kettering oncologist, Dr. Zofia Stadler, stating my termination of treatment with MSK for their *mis*treatment while I was a patient there), a lengthy account of my current struggles and the change of course I am currently pursuing, and an addendum (the Modern Hippocratic Oath).

Some good news to share with you: the raw extreme diet has fired the interest of Skyhorse Publishing (who'll publish my *Diary of a Radical Cancer Warrior* this fall 2011) to offer me a small contract to write a new book, which I have tentatively titled *Raw Extreme: Losing Weight, Self-Improvement and Changing the World While Spending Almost Nothing!*

Also, in my intention to cement my legacy, I am spending down my life's savings and self-producing a number of new CDs that will be released in 2011–2012. My website will have all of them for sale. In addition, I will be mounting new large-scale performance works for as long as I am able, including *Sweet Science Suite: A Scientific Soul Music Honoring of Muhammad Ali*, a big band-dance-video tribute to the Greatest (and we intend to have him at the world premiere!); the manga-operas *Deadly She-Wolf Assassin at Armageddon!* and *Voice of the Dragon 3: Dragon Vs. Eagle (Enter The White Barbarians)*, all of which I will self-produce.

Once again, thank you to the many friends who have contributed car rides, money, and love.

December 15, 2010

Dear Sifu (or more appropriately, Simu★) Ho,

The news recently conveyed in your e-mail is all but unbearable, yet, on some level, unsurprising. Despite not being with you for your previous heroic struggles with the capitalist-bred beast feasting on your organic cells, I could sense that this recent bout of cancer was the strongest and most vindictive, and, on some level, knew that I had met you at your paradoxically strongest and weakest state—at those rare moments in human history when the flash of genius and undiluted self-possession intersect in a person before a potentially cataclysmic event, as in the late Coltrane and Malcolm, and the handful of revolutionary spirits who have changed the world forever and shone as a beacon unto humanity. This is the Fred Ho I have had the amazing, trembling, inspiring, shaming, breathtaking, humbling, and empowering privilege to work with. It has destroyed myself and remade myself, it is destroying myself and remaking myself, it is teaching me to create myself in my own image. It is the first feeling of liberation I've ever experienced and its power makes me tremble as much as it makes me awake. It is perhaps the equivalent of what some say is finding God.

In short, the experience of working with you is not legible in the register of words. It is life incarnate that I have met in you, life-for-itself, in a way I didn't know could even exist. And trying to write about what you mean to me is perhaps an ill-guiding attempt, but remaining silent in the face of this news would be an even deeper crime. So please indulge me, in my most vain attempt, to describe my encounter with you, and how much you have meant to me.

Our meeting was almost a year ago, if you remember, on October 22, 2009, and I was in the midst of overlapping crises regarding the nature of my thesis subject. Having tapped into something I felt was there but with little inchoate literature to validate it, I was confused and felt lost: was there a relationship between jazz,

African American radicalism, and a whole epistemology with its roots in contradiction to capitalist, European ethos? Did anyone even give a shit? And who was I, white boy, to even theorize and perform such things?

And then, while walking around campus, I see a poster on a column, with none other than you, championing your Baritone Saxophone high, and above reading, "Come join us for a lecture with Revolutionary Socialist, Writer, and Baritone Saxophonist Fred Ho on "Jazz and the Revolutionary Imagination" and "The Black Arts Movement and the Asian-American Movement."

It was one of the few times I let out a roar, alone, in public. It is/ was a supreme moment of cosmic validation.

The time since then has been the most extraordinary life-changing process. I have met the most cutting-edge cultural cadre in America, and potentially on Earth. I have met Salim and his son and collaborating with each of them in their respective environments; I have borne witness to some of the most profound and revolutionary works of art ever conceived; I have read Marx with Arabelle and seen Joel Kovel speak with her and Peter, talked literature with Chong, and met the amazing and strong-willed Alice; I have become closer with Quincy and forged a stronger revolutionary bond; I have helped build and maintain a garden, I have learned how to cook.

But most of all, I have been constantly illuminated by the least compromising, most revolutionary human being I have ever met, one who lives in an age of uncompromising mediocrity and the all-but-defeat of the revolutionary left; I have seen that it is not only possible to be a lifelong activist and revolutionary matriarchal Luddite socialist—I have learned that it is the *only* possible way to live with dignity and all the personal force and power that implies.

I have learned to look at myself and see how much I lack, how much I hurt and how trapped I am in petit-bourgeois whiteness;

I have learned to shed such scales and grow a stronger, more dignified, and more loving skin.

As the caterpillar, I looked into the eyes of the butterfly. The butterfly said: there is no logical way to become butterfly. You must find the way to become the butterfly yourself. I can only inspire you, I can only show you that that butterfly exists. You must find the butterfly inside yourself.

They say the true Master is not Master over others, but Master over herself. That makes you, Fred Ho, the truest Master of all.

I feel guilty that I have not grown as much as I could have in this past year, that I have not become self-reliant, that I have not become sterling in my time and commitments, that I still engage with petit-bourgeois friends from the past that hold me back and want nothing more than me to slink into mediocrity; I feel guilty that your time on Earth is limited and I did not spend every minute of it soaking up your vast accumulated knowledge and presence.

But I also know that the forces you have helped me unlock are working their way through my body, and that soon they will explode into self-realization. I know that the lessons you have taught me but I did not fully hear will echo louder and louder until they become a symphony that surpasses the mundane and touches the sublime. I know that one day I will be an amazing composer and the best baritone saxophonist on Earth, bar none. I know that will set a revolutionary example for others to follow as you did for me, and do so at a historically critical time.

Fred, I will spend every last fiber of my being continuing the struggle to create a new society within the rotten, dying corpse of the old; I will use every cell to cleanse my body and soul of the cancers of self-obsessions, consumerism, procrastination, and self-doubt; I will use every carbon molecule to build the new Ben Barson, who truly lives up to that name, and fights uncompromisingly for dignity, liberation, and a new human. I will use every brain neuron and muscle tendon to prepare to fight in the upcoming crises Wallerstein details, in the upcoming collapse of Capitalism and its replacement with whatever hellish modification comes to surface, but will not lose the importance of what we are fighting FOR, of creating that society in the here and now; I will continue my self-revolution until I am able to be an effective revolutionary, one who understands the world they are trying to create because they have seen it inside themselves.

I will continue your struggle while remaining, and becoming, myself.

Fred Ho, I love you, so much. You are the single most influential person I have ever met. I still feel that I do not deserve to have crossed paths with you and I thank the Gods each day that we did. I hope I have honored my commitments to you as your apprentice, and I will continue your legacy in this life and the next to the best I am able. I wish you all the happiness in the world in the time you have left on Earth.

Love,

Benjamin Barson

★ *Simu* is the Chinese expression for "master/mother," a matriarchalist honorific, in contrast to the patriarchal *sifu* (master/father).

DIARY 28: THE END IS NEAR—FACING THE CROSSROADS

January 7, 2011,

Since "Diary Number 33" (November 1, 2010), every day has been a race against time, a rapid-fire succession of decisions, struggles and battles, investigation, and experiment. Accompanying this urgency has been a roller coaster of emotions that influence (for better or worse) my attitudes about my confidence to beat cancer.

The cancer war diary has been both a tool for self-reflection and self-awareness, as well as a way to share with all those who are concerned about my well-being, who want to know how I'm doing, who love and desire to support me in any way they can, as well as a way to communicate to a larger audience who might benefit from my lessons and experiences conveyed in real-time struggle.

What I'm about to present herein expresses the grave uncertainty and extremism of what might be the final stage of this war against cancer that now has spanned more than four years.

I have decided not to theorize or extrapolate lessons in this particular diary entry as I realize that answers might not be forthcoming or even possible.

I struggle every minute between having hope, confidence, and determination, to ever-increasing moments of anger, disappointment, and acceptance of a doomed inevitability. I struggle not to have negativity dominate my attitudes or decisions, not to let anger rule me, and to continually seek solutions, to allow this war to better me and not fill me with bitterness. The excitement and optimism of the new Fred Ho, toward my qualitatively better understanding of the future for revolutionary change in the world, my increased imaginative and creative abilities, the exponential improvement in my saxophone skills and artistry, in these ways, I have taken the cancer war as a gift to change me in profound personal, physical, and philosophical ways. There is no possibility of going back to a normal life, only the uncertainty, excitement and dread, of the future, but a future I am determined to live with dignity, joy, creativity, and dedicated to solutions, no matter how impossible they may seem. Cancer, in a profound irony, has become a gift of self-transformation, one I have accepted and chosen to manifest, but one that may come with the ultimate price of my death. The Samurai code says, "All warriors live as if they are preparing for death." In that way, every second alive is consummated with meaning, service, and intense confrontation of all challenges.

Writing and sharing my thoughts, feelings, and ideas with everyone who reads these diary entries has been a true therapy, indeed, the most exceptional and best form of healing and dissipation of negativity I could have found, primarily because it was self-devised, and not paid for in purchasing professional help (what I chide as the "mistreatment treatment"). Of course, practicing my saxophone daily, as I see it, is my daily form of meditation. I visualize through my sound how I want to feel, what I seek, and how I empty myself of past baggage to receive that which will come.

I begin writing this entry as another winter blizzard begins, and I reiterate in my mind how much I dislike the cold and the grayness, and visualize and seek to spend any future winters in my life in the tropics, with sun, lots of light, the ocean, and daily snorkeling and encounters with marine life.

I remain fixated upon the future, my goal to become a part-time farmer, which I believe allowed me to recover rapidly and vigorously from the seventh surgery in four years to remove the third tumor (second primary rectal cancer), in 2009, and which I still maintain (and regret) that if I had continued the farm work for 2010, may very well have obviated this recurrence, which now threatens my life in a way I feel might be the final showdown.

Second, I am intensely working to cement my legacy and producing a spate of recordings, books, and special operas for however long I have left with the energy and ability to do this life work. I am spending down every cent I have earned and saved to self-finance these projects as I am now completely done with the music business and nonprofit performing arts institutions with the exception of a small handful of curators who have shown their exceptional humanity, generosity, and support prior to and during the cancer war.

Third, I am devoting all of my energy toward a new revolutionary praxis (theory and practice), one for which the scientific soul sessions is the avatar, innovating upon an antimanifest destiny Marxism. More on this later.

And lastly, I continue to seek a deeper and more profound love in my many friendships, to make new friends, and without the possibility of employment in an academic institution, to take on students in private musical, political, and philosophical/life instruction regularly in my apartment.

NO COMPROMISE: THE EXTREME PATH TO BEATING CANCER

By October of 2010, a turn had begun in my strategy of my war against cancer. I have always recognized that I personally may not win as cancer and capitalism are inextricable, but I would have to try and set a new course with a strategy that would initiate defeating both, what I now refer to as "bringing down the matrix" (a simultaneous micro- and macro-revolutionary transformation of extrication and prefiguration—refusing to participate in the system, including its health care protocols and paradigm, and immediately begin a precursory path).

I decided to pursue a raw (or live) food therapy and postponed the mainstream industrialized medical pathway of surgery to completely remove my rectum and permanently install a colostomy bag (an irreversible procedure). I had constructed a plan to monitor the progress of the raw food therapy with three monthly ultrasound scans (which are nonradiative), the first in early November to establish a baseline measurement, the second in December to measure growth or recession, and the third, in January 2011 to have the data for a final decision about surgery.

In my plan, the possibility of surgery remained a serious option, but I wanted and needed to investigate the raw food path.

As I shared earlier, wonderful benefits quickly manifested from this course of action. I want to reinforce these changes because I resolutely believe that the raw diet is a solution to many of the problems caused by the mainstream medical treatments and offers many practical benefits to many maladies.

1. Raw extremism permanently fixed hypertension. At one time during mid-2010, my blood pressure had reached the dangerous numbers of 170/120, and the prescription medication was only making a small improvement. After two weeks on raw food, with rapid weight loss, my blood pressure reached normal (120/80). It presently is now more than perfect: 110/70.

2. Peripheral neuropathy (pain and deterioration of finer finger ability) is now gone. My saxophone technique, if I may boast, has reached a new level of virtuosity, and I am convinced that, at least technically, I am the greatest baritone saxophonist that has ever lived. There is still some slight peripheral neuropathy in my toes, but I don't use those to play the saxophone (at least not yet!).

3. Sexual functioning has improved. While I still remain unable to ejaculate, my erections are more frequent and vigorous, and my libido has improved considerably.

4. At one point, I was losing 1 pound a day without loss of appetite or quantity or quality of food I eat. I was 225 pounds midsummer 2010. I now weigh 170 pounds, losing 55 pounds in three months, with increased energy, stamina, and strength. How about that! I have had to alter all my outfits and give away many shirts and pants, punched many new belt holes, and go shopping in secondhand stores for new shirts and outer wear. This has all been fun and exciting. I am told that I have inspired many around me to at least consider, and some people have actually taken up raw-ism. I have decided that I don't want to lose any more weight so I have resumed eating some cooked foods. But a clear, definitive, and wonderful paradigm shift has happened in going raw. I have permanently turned off the gas to my stove and oven to disallow any compromise. After about twenty days of cold turkeying, the psychological addiction, and temptation to compromise and eat cooked food, I now no longer really have desire for all of what were once my favorite (cooked) foods. I can sit with friends who are eating a cooked meal, which I used to relish, and not be interested at all. Wow! Who would've thunk? I must thank my beloved friend and inspiration Peter Lew, cofounder of the

Raw Fight Club (which continues to meet Saturday evenings), who has been teacher and comrade-in-arms. Peter and my friend Tom Buckner continue to struggle with me (and I ask them to continue to tough-love me as hard as they can) to stop eating seafood (I eat a lot of raw seafood, and some cooked). They may succeed!

5. The bowel movement problems of tenesmus (the urge and feeling like I have to go to the toilet but unable to evacuate my excrement) and spasmodicity (painful, difficult, and explosive bowel movements) have been greatly reduced since going raw extreme.

6. A profound philosophical change has occurred for me, one which I believe can be the new paradigm for human society of eliminating factory farming and the system of industrialized food production (and much of industrialized medicine and culture as a whole) that relies upon, reinforces and expands the matrix of inducing false wants and needs, hype and wanton and health-destructive consumerism, and the fundamental eco-destructiveness of capitalism endemic to mass production, unlimited consumption, and waste. I now firmly and clearly see that without revolutionary Ludditism (the elimination of most industrialism), that going green and local is not only ineffective but also a Trojan horse. Self-sufficient food production by everyone or in small cooperative arrangements must replace agribusiness industrial food production. Society would be healthier, happier, and disestranged from the natural world (our denatured-ness as a result of the imperative to conquer and control nature fueled by capitalism); and the planet would not be degraded and toxic.

However, as the November ultrasound scan proved, raw could not defeat cancer. The tumor had grown about 40 percent, causing much alarm and consternation from the allopathic doctors.

I could not reject the improvements of the raw path but had to urgently consider additional pathways before the January 4, 2010, final ultrasound scan.

And after four years of what my friend Dr. Joseph Harris characterizes as me being "the perfect cancer patient" for the discipline and commitment I exerted to the allopathic paradigm, there has been no real reward to my loyalty and diligence.

True, I am still alive, that's the upside. But the downsides are many: cancer has not been eliminated, many after-problems from the draconic treatments diminished my quality of life, over $1 million has been spent, and I have lost trust, faith, confidence, and any hope for finding a solution (to an end to cancer with the allopathic paradigm for me). The fact that I'm still alive and have been able to use the cancer war for self-transformation and self-improvement came from my determination to never *be* sick (yes, I have been exhausted, suffered combat fatigue from multiple tours of duty, angry, depressed, suicidal . . .). But I never thought of myself as a sick person, never allowed myself to act as if I'm sick.

My friends have noted, even when I was very ill, mostly from the effects of surgery, radiation, and chemo, at worst, unable to be awake for more than fifteen minutes a day, that I never acted like a sick person, that even in those fifteen minutes, and used every minute to write, create, theorize, and socialize to the best that I could during the worst of the worse. For these past four years, I followed the prescription for cancer treatment, and more importantly and profoundly, I devised my own methods for recovery and solace.

THE ALLOPATHIC PROBLEM: IS IT INCOMPETEANCE, CONSPIRACY, OR JUST HOW THE SYSTEM WORKS?

In this final leg of my cancer war, even should I want to fight to keep the door open to the capitalist industrialized medicine, they have shut it for me.

I will now name names of the culprits.

Dr. Jason Bratcher of Beth Israel Hospital reneged on his agreement with me to do three ultrasound scans to assess the growth or recession of the tumor based upon my three-month trial path of raw extreme and, since early December, alternative treatment. The November test established a baseline measure of the tumor (1.8 cm ×

1.7 cm). The December scan, disappointingly, showed that the tumor had grown 40 percent (2.5 cm × 2 cm). The January test would have been my final evaluation for which I would make a final decision to do the rectal removal surgery and irreversible colostomy bag. But a few days before that test scheduled for January 4, 2011, Dr. Bratcher called me to cancel it saying he believed that such a third test would be a waste of time as he believes that surgery is the only course I should take. He was even so dishonest as to say that having three scans was not what he and I had agreed to!

While I believe his motivation and intentions were good from the point of view of his dogmatic allopathic paradigm, he violated our trust and agreement, and it felt as if he was *not* putting my wishes first and attempting to railroad me.

Out of disgust with him in particular, but for the growing arrogance of the allopathic path, I immediately called Dr. Joseph Martz of Beth Israel Hospital. Two weeks before Dr. Bratcher's cancellation, I had decided against furthering seeing Dr. Jose Guillem of MSK and had an appointment to see Dr. Joseph Martz, head of colorectal surgery at Beth Israel Hospital, where I had previously received my cancer treatments (multiple surgeries and chemo-radiation) from 2007 to the end of 2008. During the meeting with Dr. Martz, I told him I was no longer interested in returning to MSK and to Dr. Guillem in particular. Dr. Martz was curious as to why I would leave the stellar care of Guillem and the much-vaunted MSK, and I succinctly told him it was because of institutional arrogance.

During the winter holidays, apparently Dr. Bratcher had learned from Dr. Martz or somehow via the Beth Israel machinery that I had scheduled a January 20, 2011, surgery for rectal removal and colostomy installation, and Bratcher, without my permission, went ahead and cancelled the January 4, 2011, ultrasound scan. I called Bratcher's office to tell his staff that I still wanted to do the ultrasound scan, that I had *tentatively* scheduled a surgery date with Dr. Martz, but that I still had not decided to go forward with the surgery and wanted to keep the final ultrasound scan I had planned.

Now angered by Dr. Bratcher's betrayal and the increasing suspicion I was having of an allopathic conspiracy to railroad me into doing this surgery, I called Dr. Martz and instructed him to cancel the surgery because I was disgusted with their system of medicine and the imperious attitudes of everyone in this system in their disregard of a patient's (my) wishes.

With only one business day available before the New Year's holiday break, I scrambled to get another appointment for that same day of January 4, but no longer at Beth Israel, now at NewYork-Presbyterian/Weill Cornell Hospital radiology.

They scheduled me late in the day on December 30 (a Thursday) for Tuesday, January 4. I spent the New Year's weekend believing that I was going to have an ultrasound scan.

Late in the business day of Monday, January 3, 2011, NewYork-Presbyterian/Weill Cornell leaves a phone message saying that the ultrasound scan for the next morning had to be cancelled due to some vague scheduling error.

Angered again, I call and have it rescheduled to January 11, 2011, with profuse apologies from their representative.

Late in the afternoon on January 10, 2011, I get a message left on my answering machine that they were canceling the January 11, 2011, scan, leaving no reason for doing this.

At that point, I was burning with anger. It was now after the close of business. I called them and left a tirade on their voice mails.

The allopathic industry had made the decision for me. I am now committed to abandon their methods completely, though I still find their diagnostic tools in their paradigm to be still useful, namely, colonoscopy and ultrasound scan (which does not use radiation).

The slew of CT-PT scans, CEA, and blood work tests during the entire past four years had shown I was cancer free, in remission, but clearly I wasn't, and it was only my own keen sense about myself did I always and accurately know that I had cancer time and time again. The allopathic oncologists all admit that their toolbox of expensive and draconic treatments had not completely gotten rid of cancer.

ANGER AND ANXIETY

Anger toward the allopathic medical establishment resulted in my sending this letter to my family and some of my closest friends on January 11, 2011:

Dear family and friends,

The U.S. mainstream medical establishment has forced me now completely reject them. The ultrasound scan I was scheduled for today to ascertain the success or failure of my alternative plan to defeat cancer was cancelled. This has easily made the choice for, even though I up until this, was still seriously considering their proposed treatment of radical surgery. The cancellation of this third and final scan by Dr. Bratcher violated the agreement we made in order to railroad me into the surgery.

Even with this offense, I immediately scrambled to get the scan done by New York Presbyterian/Cornell Weil, but due to their incompetence, they called me at 3:30pm yesterday, just as I was about to do the enema prep, to say they won't do the scan because it was misscheduled. For a moment, I was very angry, but I took a Zen moment to breathe and reflect: the maker-of-the-universe has sent me a message to commit to my rejection of mainstream medicine.

The decision is done. After another attempt to reschedule, I will do the scan on Monday, January 11, 2011, but that will not affect any decision anymore. I believe having information is still important. But I am now thoroughly and completed done with the U.S. medical industry. It has been an abject failure. It offers no solutions. I will find the solution on my own and with help of those who understand and support my decision. Those who do not, please do not obstruct or interfere.

I have cancelled my treatment (more mistreatment) by Memorial Sloan-Kettering. I have cancelled my secondary insurance with United Healthcare because I detest the insurance industry completely. I only retain Medicare, a single-payer, which I believe should be the right of all Americans. I can only participate in things that I believe in. To ask me to be a compromiser goes against everything I am. You might as well ask me to commit suicide.

I no longer have anger, only dedication and focus to truly beat cancer. I will get that miracle because that is what I am meant to do.

Love,

FRED

My youngest sister Flora had an e-mail exchange during this time. She asked me if I was clear about what to expect in facing death and the long-expected suffering I will face if cancer progresses. Here is what I wrote to her:

Dear Flora,

In the past four years, I have been surrounded by terminal cancer patients, and at my alternative doctor's office, daily see people with stage 4 metastatic cancer, tremendous suffering but who are relieved by Dr. Akpinar. I have been through hell and back several times and almost committed suicide.

I subscribe to euthanasia. I will know when I have truly lost, and I won't be a drain, burden, or imposition upon anyone.

I am for the first time in the cancer war, truly free and feel great because I'm in charge.

As Dr. Harris said, I was the perfect cancer patient: did everything the allopathic program told me to do, was disciplined, didn't complain, did research and educated myself, built a support network, etc. As I see it now, they failed because they cannot think beyond their training and their paradigms. My case is so unusual that it *demands* and *necessitates* thinking outside of the box. Going to the farm was my idea and because I didn't do that in 2010, and because I didn't commit to raw food, I am in the trouble that I am in now *but no one* on the allopathic side could have instructed me in this. The farm did several things:

1. increased nutritional density;
2. natural mineral water from the ground;
3. vitamin D from sunshine;
4. higher altitude (1,000 feet above sea level) oxygenation;
5. sweat therapy which naturally rid my body of toxins, including massive chemo drugs while I worked daily on the land.

I didn't go far enough with the farm. I should have gone 100% raw and I *know* that I would not have gotten cancer again. The cancer came back because of the tenesmus, the putrification of my feces being lodged in my anus. That caused it in 2008 (the second primary) and it caused the recurrence. When I asked the oncologist to opine about my theory, all she could say was, "It could be." They don't know and they don't bother to know.

I only want solutions now. Nothing less.

Love,

FRED

THE START OF A SOLUTION: FINDING A TRUE PEOPLE'S PHYSICIAN

By early December 2010, upon the repeated offering of Mike Byfield, I went to see a good friend of his who is an alternative doctor. Two years ago, Mike had recommended that I go see him, but two years ago, I was still the perfect, dutiful cancer patient to the capitalist industrialized medical establishment (CIME, rhymes with "slime" or "crime") and dismissed most of the alternative pathways as unscientific, unverifiable, and profiteers in a New Age guise.

Reluctantly, and skeptically, I set up an appointment with Dr. Bluten (Bill) Akpinar, and an Access-A-Ride transport to his office at the very edge of Queens, Long Island, for December 7, 2010.

Here's what little I knew about Dr. Akpinar before I visited him: while a dentist, he was one of the first to oppose mercury fillings and removed them from patients' teeth. During the 1990s, when his girlfriend had been diagnosed with cervical cancer, he began seeking solutions that led him to ozone treatments. It has been almost two decades, and she has been cancer free, though from what I learned speaking with her, it took about eighteen months before the cancer disappeared, along with supplement saturation and changes to her diet.

Dr. Akpinar's office is in a three-story home, which he used to reside in, very unlike the institutionalized buildings of mainstream doctor offices and hospitals.

The first thing I noticed upon sitting in the patient's waiting area was how cheerful and optimistic all the patients were. They were joking, openly discussing their medical struggles, including serious injuries, constant pain issues, and even more advanced cancer and maladies than my own.

Dr. Akpinar himself is a force of nature, full of good, effervescent energy and wellness projected toward his patients. I explained to him how the allopathic medical establishment didn't give me any chances, and he obstreperously remarked in his palpable disgust with the CIME, that he is given the discarded patients, the ones for whom establishment medicine has forsaken. He immediately took me to the various small rooms and showed me his treatment methods. I met a sixty-three-year-old black woman suffering from stage 4 colon cancer that had metastasized to her liver. I watched as Dr. Bill (as he is fondly called) injects her with ozone. This was an eye-opener for me, watching her skin actually bubble from these infusions inside her veins. He then proceeded to do the same for me, and so, I now began my new path that has since included an array of treatments, including shark cartilage (sharks are the only animal on this planet that don't seem to get cancer), vitamin B_{12}, acupuncture to remove the blockages and obstructions to my circulation and flow of chi energy, sweat therapy in the small sauna (Dr. Akpinar claims to have written "the book" on sweat therapy, including having published *No Sweat, Know Sweat*), ozone infusions, and hyperbaric chamber (laying a small submarine like chamber of increased pressure to compress the oxygen and ozone into my tissue), and other applications.

Dr. Akpinar is the closet embodiment to the great people's doctor and legendary martial artist Wong Fei-hung. Of Turkish descent, he trained in alternative medicine in China (as well as martial arts) and goes to China twice annually. But more significantly, unlike others in the alternative wellness industry, and certainly starkly different from anyone in the allopathic industrialized medicine, after I explained my current situation of living on federal disability and having been financially nongainful for four years, he agreed to treat me based upon whatever I can pay. (Note: I am hesitant to recount this, as I do *not* want readers to believe that the same arrangement will always hold for others.)

How about that? In my appreciation and gratitude, since I have lost fifty-five pounds in these past three months, I have given to him and his staff various original jackets I have designed and owned, made from Chinese and Japanese fabrics, since they don't fit me anymore. Everyone, including Dr. Bill, truly loves these couture gifts from me. As he exclaimed, "This man [Fred] has literally given me the shirt off his back. What more gratitude can I be given?"

I now go three times a week for all-day treatments. My entire Tuesdays, Thursdays, and Saturdays are spent there. I feel amazingly well, energized and more importantly, happy and optimistic about beating cancer. I don't feel like leaving Dr. Bill's office. I never feel that way coming from mainstream medical appointments. Just the opposite: I am invariably angry or depressed after those appointments, tests, and treatments, and want to get the hell out of these places as fast as I can!

I have come to realize that CIME doctors focus upon medicine, while healers, like Dr. Bill, focus upon humans.

We'll see if this path will beat cancer or not. But on this path, I feel that I'm finally in control, my dignity respected, and my well-being listened to and appreciated.

The quality of my life has significantly improved in this short period. I am in the best shape of my entire life, feeling like I am twenty-one years ago (Dr. Akpinar's fourth and most recent book, *Priceless Prescriptions*, is a basic and usefully primer for wellness, health, and antiaging principles). If cancer is to take my life, at least during this period, I have found a new and profound improvement to my quality of life I never imagined could be possible, with equally profound side effects that have included excelling in my saxophone playing, creative and imaginative surges and new vistas, soaring happiness and love, and finally, a confidence in my struggle to beat cancer, and an attendant happiness and joy.

I still live every day as if preparing for death. But my attitude and energy is not about cynicism, anger, depression, or testiness, which has been generated by the nonsolutions and institutional arrogance of the capitalist industrial medical establishment.

A GREAT DAY IN LONDON: DECEMBER 9, 2010

I now rarely watch television, completely repulsed by the sophomoric, stultifying, and imbecilic shows, but I do watch network evening news to get the point of view of the corporate media about society and the world.

During the time of November through December 2011, I waged battle after battle with the capitalist industrial medical machine, accounted above. Typically, I am either angry, depressed, or both after dealing with the machine, from coming out a doctor's appointment, to having a test done, to the moribund environment of antiseptic and dehumanized waiting rooms. Even the expensive office architecture of Memorial Sloan-Kettering designed by the top dollar-fetching architect Maya Lin, with its predictable light flowing gentle waterfalls, bonsai trees, and Zen-like stone pools, exude the perfunctory professionalism ("have a nice day") and superficial pretense toward "caring" of crass medical profiteering and institutional arrogance and self-importance.

So, after a long day of combined anger and anxiety generated by the affronting institutional arrogance of MSK, I turn on the nightly network news on Friday, December 9, 2010, and see a London riot by youth engaged at exorbitantly escalating costs of education, storming and overcoming the security assigned to Prince Charles and Camilla, scaring the shit out of the two royals, and I get a delicious sense of euphoric satisfaction! What a great day in London! Right on, scare the shit out of those parasites! I remember during the darkest days of my chemo hammering how I watched documentaries of Muhammad Ali, the true people's champion, to inspire and fire my fighting spirit, to rejoice in retribution, to celebrate the upsurges of underdogs, and to relish revolutionary redemption. Hoorah!

One day, the Goliath of insurance company-dominated profiteering megamedicine will be toppled and destroyed by the slingshot-wielding David.

Concurrently, on that same NBC-TV news show, chief medical correspondent Dr. Nancy Schneidermann reported what has been confirmed for nearly half a century: that of the seven thousand chemicals in cigarettes, seven hundred cause cancer. And millions in the matrix continue to smoke.

LIGHTNESS OF WEIGHT, LIGHTNESS OF BEING

The decision to forego another surgery, to proceed full force in an alternative direction (though admittedly since using capitalist medicine's diagnostic tools of colonoscopies and ultrasound scans, while rejecting the high radiation PT/CT scans), has generated an unexpected but revelatory lightness of being about me and in my soul.

I have left mainstream medicine for good. I have left the music and nonprofit arts industry for good. I no longer will partake in anything that is not firmly committed to integrity, imagination, and excellence. So I gladly and easily rejected exploitative and disrespectful offers by Starkland Records, the Hitchcock Institute of American Music at Brooklyn College (for a project celebrating the East, a black cultural nationalist/pan-Africanist independent institution of the late 1960s–early 1980s, an idea I initiated, and for which I supplied many of the program ideas and speaker contacts) and the East Coast Asian Student Union keynote conference speaker (a network for which I was one of the original founders and organizers in 1978), a silly invitation by the Harvard Asian American law school students conference to speak on a panel about Asian Americans in the "entertainment business," etc. To quote the ingenious impresario Marty Khan, "My second favorite word is 'no.'"

Meanwhile, I gladly and enthusiastically accepted offers from Teatro Vida and Amherst Community Television to host a special manga/book-CD reception for a new release in April, to serve on a National Endowment for the Arts panel, to reschedule a performance with Dr.

Salim Washington (our Afro Asian scientific soul duo) in Troy, New York, for spring 2011, to speak at a Cal Massey tribute concert at the University of Connecticut–Storrs, and the great honor facilitated by composer-friend Charles Wuorinen to accept a commission from the Boston Symphony Orchestra to compose a short work, *Fanfare to Stop the Creeping Meatball!*, for the 2011 Tanglewood Music Festival.

LISTENING TO WHAT THE MAKER OF THE UNIVERSE IS INSTRUCTING

The CIME shut the door on me, though their door remains open if I submit and concede to their paradigm and protocols, and of course, pay abundantly for their services. I remain an atheist, and still, with strong resistance on my part, am not big on spirituality. But I realize that somehow, in the four years of this brutal cancer war, that a force has been acting on my behalf, not allowing me to be randomized in the clinical trial for the superdrug Avastin (which would have surely worsened my quality of life or killed me, or I would have committed suicide from such worsening); getting me to work on the farm during mid-2009; to the present, having the door close upon me by blocking my ultrasound scans and making me to commit to a completely nonallopathic path. The Maker of the Universe is always telling us, but are we open or capable of hearing? I have now reached the point of struggling and seeking to hear.

A TIDBIT AS TO WHY INDUSTRIO-TECHNO-CENTRISM CREATES MORE PROBLEMS THAN IT SOLVES

On January 6, 2011, Dr. Nancy Snyderman, chief medical correspondent for NBC-TV, reported that the Department of Health and Human Services has ordered the Food and Drug Administration to address the problem that 41 percent of American youth between the ages of twelve to fifteen years old have dental fluorosis, an irreversible condition caused by excessive ingestion of fluoride in public drinking water. *Irreversible!*

DIARY 29: LETTER TO DR. ZOFIA STADLER REGARDING MY TERMINATION OF TREATMENT AT MEMORIAL SLOAN-KETTERING

January 19, 2011

Dear Dr. Stadler,

I am writing personally to you because you are the only person at Memorial Sloan-Kettering that I respect and like anymore.

Perhaps this is because you came up in Canada and have a heart about medicine not poisoned by the American medical system.

I am notifying you that I am discontinuing as a patient of Memorial Sloan-Kettering due to the insulting and offensive institutional arrogance of MSK, from the staff to the nurses to Doctors Guillem, Herr, Toujier, to the psychiatrist who met me regarding suicide counseling, etc.

In my pursuit of alternative treatment, beginning with the raw-food therapy and now involving ozone and acupuncture, I feel the best I have ever felt and solved every single side effect caused by the massive amounts of surgeries, chemotherapies, and radiation I faced for four years. I am still working on hydronephrosis, but I have no urological problems once I rejected the proposed treatments by Drs. Herr and Toujier in your urology department.

No one at MSK has ever offered any of these considerations that have dramatically improved the quality of my life and have almost fixed every problem as an outcome of the draconic and severe treatments I have received in the past four years.

Here is a brief historical detail of what has led me to reject MSK, a more detailed open letter to the entire institution, including its CEO and board of directors, will be forthcoming.

1. Dr. Guillem at our last and final meeting, after I waited for five hours in the waiting area (and I don't fault anyone for this), met me for five minutes (I knew he had a long and exasperating day)—and charged me over $300 for five minutes of no information—to tell my sister, who is a doctor, when she asked him, "What are Fred's curative chances if he does the surgery you are proposing," he replied, sitting smugly arms folded across his chest, "I don't know." He provided no explanation to my question as to why a trans-anal excision could not be considered. All he said in an imperious tone, was "You can go find someone else who'll do that, but I won't." (Later, Dr. Martz, Chief Surgeon of Beth Israel gave me an explanation for my case and the prevailing thought against another trans-anal excision.). Dr. Guillem said he would not sit there or spend any time with me, my lover, and my sister on the speaker phone, and try to convince me about surgery.

   Well, if that is his attitude, why would I proceed? Simply because of his supposed expertise? After all, he excised the T1 rectal tumor, and it came back as a T3. What confidence should I have that he can even eliminate cancer for the T3?

2. None of the CT, CEA, or blood work tests showed that the rectal cancer had returned. It was confirmed on September 24, 2007 upon my expression that I believed/felt it had returned. Dr. Guillem did a digital exam and a sigmoidoscopy. He refused to prescribe to me an ultrasound scan, saying all he needed to know was that I had cancer, nothing more. He then billed me for an ultra sound scan, which has been reversed after my challenge to it to your billing department, who confirmed that indeed, no such test was done.

3. I almost committed suicide after the trans-anal excision of February 2009 when Dr. Guillem did not call me or even check on me after the surgery. I only learned two weeks later in a follow up visit that he was not able to sew me up from too much scar tissue. During that time of unknown, I faced brutal pain and could not sleep for twelve days and twelve nights. That was tantamount to torture.

   Now in October 2010 with this recurrence, I therefore cancelled the surgery, though I had not removed it as an option, and thus devised my own plan of procedure.

4. Drs. Herr and Toujier never saw me before the February 2009 surgery, never spoke to me, never followed up with me, never returned my calls.

5. I could never get a doctor at MSK to ever return my phone call and speak to me directly for the entire duration I have been a patient at MSK. I could never have the expectation that I could speak to a doctor when I needed or wanted to. This is inexcusable.

6. You stated to me that you and Dr. Guillem, my principal doctors at MSK, rarely ever talk, much less meet, so presumably, details of my case and health are never collaboratively discussed or examined.

Because of my respect *only* for you, I am always happy to have a conversation with you.

Sincerely,

FRED HO

Finally, in this series of cancer war diary entries, I am including below the modern Hippocratic Oath, which only Dr. Bill boldly displays and exhibits, both in his book, as well as in his being. I would opine that most CIME doctors couldn't even recite, much less summarize, espouse, and practice any of these principles. The CIME doctors and staff are prisoners of their paradigm, protocols, and the profit-driven system. Note at the end that the greatest reward for a healer is not money, career, status, but life and art. That should be the reward for all of us: to have a true life fixated upon healing and improvement for people and sublime creativity, beauty, and the journey of imagination.

THE MODERN HIPPOCRATIC OATH

I swear to fulfill to the best of my ability and judgment, this covenant:

I will respect the hard-won scientific gains of those physicians in whose steps I walk and gladly share such knowledge as is mine with those who are to follow.

I will apply, for the benefit of the sick, all measures [that] are required, avoiding those twin traps of overtreatment and therapeutic nihilism.

I will remember that there is art to medicine as well as science, and that warmth, sympathy, and understanding may outweigh the surgeon's knife or the chemist's drug.

I will not be ashamed to say "I know not," nor will I fail to call in my colleagues when the skills of another are needed for a patient's recovery.

I will respect the privacy of my patients, for their problems are not disclosed to me that the world may know. Most especially must I tread with care in matters of life and death. If it is given to me to save a life, all thanks. But it may also be within my power to take a life; this awesome responsibility must be faced with great humbleness and awareness of my own frailty. Above all, I must not play at God.

I will remember that I do not treat a fever chart, a cancerous growth, but a sick human being, whose illness may affect the person's family and economic stability. My responsibility includes these related problems, if I am to care adequately for the sick.

I will prevent disease whenever I can, for prevention is preferable to cure.

I will remember that I remain a member of society, with special obligations to all my fellow human beings, those sound of mind and body as well as the infirm.

If I do not violate this oath, may I enjoy life and art, respected while I live and remembered with affection thereafter. May I always act so as to preserve the finest traditions of my calling and may I long experience the joy of healing those who seek my help.

DIARY 30: WE'RE GONNA DANCE! PUTTING THE STARE ON CANCER AND CONFRONTING THE TERATOGENIC-CARCINOGENIC-IOTROGENIC MATRIX!

February 24, 2011

After filing a complaint with the New York State Attorney General Office against Manhattan Diagnostic Radiology, I finally received my endo-rectal (also referred to as transanal) ultrasound scan.

What was a simple, noninvasive, nonradiological out-patient test that lasted about ten minutes, with no anesthesia administered, took over eleven days for me to get the results, and only after stomping on them repeatedly after their recurrent lies and obfuscations.

More important than the test results, which I will share below, is the lesson of this experience. Once a patient decides to not play ball with the U.S. mainstream medical establishment, as I have chosen to do, then that patient becomes pariah. In the last entry I recounted the problems and difficulties made by the CIME in blocking my self-initiated monitoring of the latest tumor. Leaving Memorial Sloan-Kettering, New York, Presbyterian/Cornell-Weill, and Beth Israel Medical Center, I found a private firm, MDR, for which I had set up an appointment, gotten my primary care doctor's prescription, and was willing to pay for out of pocket. The test did occur, but after eleven days and repeated phone calls and, finally, filing the complaint did I get Dr. Elias Kazam to complete the report and authorize its issuance. But again, they wanted to send it *only* to my doctor, not to me, which I charged violated my Patient Bill of Rights, which entitles me to all of my medical records and reports upon request.

The excuse (or what they would state is their "explanation") for the delay, as conveyed to me by Karen Kaplan of MDR, a self-admitted go-between whose job is to smooth things over, was that I should be grateful that such a brilliant doctor as Dr. Kazam was taking his time to carefully review my test, and that he usually takes longer to make his reports.

I rebutted her by stating that before scheduling the test, during the test, and after the test, I had inquired as to when I would get the report, and repeatedly told two to three business days following the procedure. Furthermore, I never requested Dr. Kazam, and since I'm fighting the fourth bout with cancer in four years, any delay worsens my prospects for any treatment decisions I would have to make. (Of course, I didn't tell her that I was devising my own treatment and no longer participated in mainstream oncology.)

Here are the results: the tumor has changed shape. Previously, measured in early December 2010, it was 2.3 cm × 2.0 cm, or roundish, it is now 3.7 cm long but 1.6 cm wide, more elongated. What seems promising though is that the tumor is punctuated. I showed the test result to a colleague of my alternative doctor who noticed this fact. Though uncertain what this means, we are hopeful that the tumor is being "squeezed" and punctuated and is retreating or dying in some parts.

My decision now is to find another place to do another ultrasound scan in two to three months.

But the lesson is clear: CIME is set up, as a system, to obviate self-healing by the patient, requiring procedural protocols and authorizations that can only be done through their system.

Self-healing invariably requires either discarding that system totally, or subterfuge and subversion of it, with many difficulties that take time, effort, and energy.

BECOMING A ZEN SPIRITUAL WARRIOR

This is what Dr. Akpinar, my alternative doctor, says we patients must become in order to fight to both the illness and the system, which I contend is synonymous.

In the 1974 historic Rumble in the Jungle boxing match, Muhammad Ali, allowed to return to boxing after being stripped of his Heavyweight Champion of the World title for refusing to be inducted into the U.S. military to fight in Vietnam (as well as being heftily fined and serving prison time), faced at-the-time current title holder the *uber-juggernaut* George Foreman. Everyone in the boxing establishment

believed Foreman would decimate the older Ali, regarded then as a has-
been from years away from the sport. However, Ali had become beloved
by the people of the world, especially the oppressed, for his courage
and defiance against U.S. imperialism. And the people were routing for
Muhammad, against the boxing establishment certainties.

Writer Norman Mailer, attending this historic fight at ringside,
remarked how Ali, in his opinion, was trying to psyche himself to go
up against the more powerful Foreman, by bodaciously shouting to the
crowd, "We're gonna dance! We're gonna dance!" over and over again.
When the two boxers faced off in the ring as the referee was issuing
instructions, Mailer remarked how Ali was putting a stare on Foreman.

After recently reviewing footage from this event, I believe that we
cancer warriors must put a stare on cancer and dance it to death.

We must have no fear, and we must have tremendous fun in
the fight against both the cancer and the CIME. We cannot let our
emotions, especially anger, which has plagued me, to rule, or we'll rue
its effects. We must use the rope-a-dope that Ali, the trickster, used to
defeat Foreman: turn the power and might of the CIME against itself,
never the while losing faith in ourselves.

More and more as I continue on the alternative path, I recognize
that allopathic practitioners (from the doctors to the staff to even the
go-betweens) might have good intentions and mean well, but they are
prisoners of a paradigm, or a system, that makes us, the cancer patients
or fighters, sicker. In my specific case, after four years of being the
perfect cancer patient, allopathic medicine now can offer no solutions,
just more of the same, though even they admit their toolbox is reduced
as radiation and chemo are now off the table given the toxification
of my left kidney and the very great risks to toxification to my only
remaining right kidney.

When I told Dr. Martz, chief colorectal surgeon at Beth Israel,
that I was refusing the surgery and pursuing alternative therapies, he
quipped, "In 2011 in New York City, this is how your cancer is treated:
surgery." The data and "evidence" for anything alternative is not within
their purview as no tests or studies on such treatments are typically
funded, so such data and evidence doesn't "exist." I subscribed to this
paradigm, as you have read in these diaries between 2006–2008. It is
not profitable to fund tests or trials on methods in which little or no

profits can be derived. After more than $1 million of treatments, tests, and examinations, I still have cancer. Clearly, there is something wrong with the paradigm.

If it is all explained as genetics, then I might as well commit suicide upon diagnosis, because that determinism of my fate precludes any possibility for intervention, only the possibility for management, which is a passive death anyways.

LOVE IN THE TIME OF SCOUNDRELS

I recently learned the term *iatrogenic*, defined as "caused by doctors" and commonly referring to "inadvertent" death or harm caused by allopathic prescription, policy, or practice (i.e., harm or death caused by medical malpractice, mistreatment, or neglect). My friend, the great poet Genny Lim, noted in an e-mail to me:

Dear Fred,

I've followed your cancer diaries for the last four years and have, like so many of your friends, marveled at your resilience, courage, prolific, creative output and determination to beat cancer. I don't blame you for giving up on industrialized medicine and the whole capitalistic system in which it operates. They have put profits, or as you term, industrialized capitalist medicine, before 'people.' It's almost as if patients are there to serve the science, not the other way around. I've heard and experienced so many horror stories about mistreatments, misdiagnosis and systemic errors, big and small, which is why malpractice insurance is so high, further driving up costs. I was scammed last year by a fake health insurance company and wound up taking my case to Consumer Watch on Channel Five.

As for medical care, I know two elderly people, my mother for one, who died of staph infections, while convalescing in hospitals. Hospitals don't like to report the high number of staph-related deaths and epidemics that occur on a regular basis. As well as the botched procedures. My daughter's boyfriend's doctor, left a portion of a hypodermic needle in his neck and even though they reassured him that the bit wouldn't pose any problems, 50 percent of his neck movement is gone and now with physical therapy he's slowly increased movement to 70%. Even the Stanford specialists were unable to help him and all covered for the first doctor's error, refusing to attribute any blame to him.

Capitalism and corporate medicine have probably killed more people than the wars in Iraq and Afghanistan put together. Western medicine is good at cutting people up, but definitely not at preventive medicine. I, myself, have gone back to eastern medicine, even though most insurance doesn't cover it. The U.S. system is paternalistic and its approach is invasive.

I'm very relieved and happy that you're now under the care of a terrific doctor, who treats and respects you as a whole person, rather than as a sick patient. Your last letter sounds much more relaxed, cheerful and hopeful, compared to the two diary entries, which chronicle your disappointment and outrage at the doctors' refusal to respect your wishes for the ultrasound test. It sounded like a cynical economic decision on their parts.

Cancer is a complex disease and the jury is still out on whether raw foods would've cured you completely or not. My Tibetan doctor recommends elimination of starch and raw foods for a "cold kidney," akin to a diabetic condition so it's hard to say if the raw diet works for every person or condition. You've been the best advocate and facilitator of your own healing so I won't be surprised if you do wind up bucking the odds again. You've still got a lot of creativity to explore so I know you'll make the best of your time on this planet, while you're still here with us. Just remember to take time out to chill!

Love in the time of capitalist scoundrels!

GENNY

Iatrogenic death in the U.S. medical system has probably killed more Americans than have the bombs and bullets of so-called terrorists in Iraq and Afghanistan annually. That is the terrorism perpetrated in the name of medicine and good intentions. As Dr. Joel Kovel told me, iatrogenic deaths are the fourth leading cause of deaths in the United States, after automobiles, heart disease, and cancer.

You are now hearing these opinions from me, who, if you've been reading these cancer war diaries, believed in and followed the mainstream medical prescriptions loyally, faithfully, and diligently.

What I am struggling with is not to let anger from feelings of disappointment, frustration, and dejection with the CIME rule and ruin me.

Therefore, I must make jest of, have fun with, and entertain myself, being one of the many Davids with my slingshot of intelligence, creativity, and spiritual power, taking on the Goliath of cancer and capitalism.

Seeing so many patients in Dr. Akpinar's office, all of us now discards and rejected by or rejecting the CIME, we empower one another sharing our experiences and experiments.

I have added now a new principle to the strategy of nutrition, hydration, oxygenation, and love, devised during the 2006–2008 period of this war: *self-healing*. We only truly heal this way. And the hope, if one is to subscribe to this power, resides in the power of one's own spirit and where-with-all to devise one's own self-healing strategies.

Mainstream medicine is the succubus. While you are in repose, believing it to be there for your best interests, it is in reality functioning according to its own logic, which inevitably is to facilitate the interests of capitalism (profits), all the while convincing you, along with its practitioners (many of whom are well intentioned), that it is healing you when indeed it is not and, often, making you sicker. Part of that succubus syndrome is increasing your dependency and debt (financial, psychological, emotional) to it.

Here is what many of the alternative folks don't want to hear: while healing must eliminate self-immolating anger and rage, to truly heal, one must eliminate financial profiteering from health, wellness, and healing; and so all of us must become in multiple and varied ways self-healers. So, too, must society restore the commons, eliminate the enclosures, and ensure self-sufficiency and end exploitation forever.

MY TREATMENT DAYS BECOME MY WELLNESS-FOCUS DAYS

Every Tuesdays, Thursdays, and Saturdays I spend all day at Dr. Akpinar's for treatments, many of which I cannot discuss herein because they, frankly, are unconventional! Should these therapies be known and adopted by many (namely by patients and some open-minded and truly concerned physicians not totally contained by capitalist interests), the entire system of medicine would be revolutionized. The verdict is still out on many of these therapies because this system will not support the kind of research and study needed to evaluate their efficacy and applicability.

On these days, I devote the minute I awake in the morning, in addition to my daily routine of hydration, herbal consumption (more below on this), daily bike riding and walks, mostly raw food meals, to include enema, exercise (isometrics), wheatgrass, and other juices, special research into other possible treatments, such as Miatake D-fraction, MMS, Johanna Budwig's organic flaxseed oil and low-fat cottage cheese protocol, vitamin D, etc.

I am constantly sifting through a lot of the alternative profiteers, since I am now convinced that health, wellness, and healing are the antithesis to commercialism and wealth accumulation.

Also on my wellness days, I pay attention to my plants, giving them my care.

As part of spending down and preparing for my death (whenever that may be), I am giving away a lot of personal belongings and money, but more importantly, my experience, knowledge, and creativity. Many people who have recently entered my orbit on this planet have greatly benefited from the range of offerings I have, from musical and artistic, to fighting the cancer war (some of Dr. Akpinar's other patients), to revolutionaries who want to make a new society.

I share my research with Dr. Akpinar and his staff, whose own modalities include hyperbaric chamber, heat or sweat therapy, shark cartilage, five mushroom serum (with the inflammatory Serapin), etc.

But the new thing that I have really, I believe, struck gold with is chaparral, a desert plant commonly found in the southwest of the United States. (I get it from Rose Mountain Herbs in New Mexico, all organic, found for me by the beautiful Charlene Muhammad, a kind and informed alternative holistic herbalist in the Baltimore area). Chaparral is very controversial. Used for a long time by Native Americans as a cancer fighter, some mainstream doctors began administering it to their patients who had nothing to lose (meaning that mainstream medicine had nothing to offer them anymore), with remarkable results. At one point, and I haven't verified this, chaparral was banned and made illegal, for risk to liver toxicity.

I drink it regularly, about two to three times a day, as a tea (both hot and cold), often while eating, as the taste is very strong and bitter. But I have gained tremendous wellness since I began using it, which started the afternoon after this last ultrasound scan, as my ten-pound box of organic dried chaparral leaf arrived later that afternoon. I can't verify its effects yet upon the cancer tumor and will do so once I get the next scan done two to three months from now. But already, I feel tremendously rejuvenated, with improved effects upon my bowel movements, surge of strength, energy and stamina, and general invigoration to my overall health. I have given bags of it to others, as I encourage and extol it.

I am searching for a very special oncologist, as I must have one to order tests and advise me on the ontology of cancer. But I am now clear as to what such an oncologist must possess:

1. Acceptance that I'm in charge
2. Openness to research and investigate all alternative treatments
3. Committed to my dignity and quality of life no matter what
4. Who won't charge me if s/he can't tell me anything I don't know or can do anything that will work

If you know of an oncologist who qualifies, by all means, let me know!

As part of my aspiring Luddite ways (yes, for you cynics, I am still word processing these diaries on a computer and distributing them via the Internet), I am endeavoring to not use plastic as much as I can. I carry liquids in glass bottles and containers, my food in linen bags and recycled wood cigar boxes, always constantly figuring out how a life without plastics can happen here and now (the one difficulty is electronics, but then, I'm trying to minimize my usage of anything electromagnetic, preferring to do most of my work with natural sunlight at sunrise until sunset, and hanging out at my local restaurant EAT, which uses candlelight on the tables, to socialize before I go to bed.

As always, the Maker of the Universe has brought offerings to me. My friends Victoria Maldonado and Mario Murillo have loaned to me their biomat and regularly supply me with well water from their farm home, carried over to me in a large milk crate of empty glass bottles when they come to the city. I sleep on the biomat nightly. The biomat is a crystal heat-therapy mattress, for which there are two used in Dr. A's facility.

Recently, friends who are independent documentary filmmakers approached me to see if I would consent to their making a film about my life and journey in this world titled *Diary of the Dragon: The (R) Evolution of Fred Ho*. Go to www.diaryofthedragon.com. They could use your support, especially financial donations.

On January 24, 2011, my latest CD featuring the Green Monster Big Band, *Year of the Tiger*, was released and can be purchased at www. bigredmediainc.com or at the Internet outlets.

And the Green Monster Big Band, conducted by my composition student Ms. Whitney George completed the "Sweet Science Suite" opus. Engineer Jon Rosenberg believes it to be my masterpiece. He describes it as "a long-lost super-baroque blaxploitation soundtrack." Since it is a homage to Muhammad Ali, it evokes much of the spirit of the 1960s and 1970s and with a revolutionary Afro Asian futurism. It will be out mid-2011 to coincide with the world premiere full-stage production of this work, which we hope the Greatest will grace us with his presence.

If I had done the surgery that many of the allopathic advocates wanted this past late October, I would not have been strong enough of body or spirit to make this recording. Jon Rosenberg is correct, as I, too, believe it to be my crowning musical work. It also introduces the young Ben Barson, my baritone saxophonist protégé, this being his debut professional recording, and he is a behemoth!

Soon, I will go snorkeling somewhere for a break and devising plans to return to working on a farm for the warmer months of this year. *Raw spring days are near.*

A good friend, Professor Beth Cleary of St. Paul, Minnesota, sent me this e-mail, as many of you have been sending me your love and support for my completely naturopathic direction.

Dear Fred:

I was thinking about you this morning (as I do many times during many days)—and then came the latest Cancer War Diary posting. When I was thinking of you I was especially heart-sore about how cruel the (human being) doctors have been with you, refusing the final ultrasounds that had been scheduled seemingly just for spite, lying, avoiding and clearly showing contempt for the alternatives you're pursuing. It's sad for all of us, as you know, that doctors at these supposedly world-class leading medical institutions are finally enclosed in brick walls, and if their methods fail and all they can do is re-prescribe the same terrible treatments and one asks, instead, for creativity and collaboration on alternatives, one slams into those brick walls. Mostly I was thinking about the courage it takes to let fear — cousin of courage — take a seat in your living room, and breathe with it. Because being kicked off the very tests which would at least have given you some baseline information as you carry forth with your own plan surely opened the door for fear. Your recent letter to the Good Doctor at Memorial Sloan-Kettering, which Ann (i.e., Ann T. Greene) posted this morning, is right on. I look forward to reading the one you're slowly but surely composing to the Whole System of MSK. They, whoever they are, need to hear from someone, you, who is actually having to walk this path. Clearly their urge is to dismiss you as a nut and add a few more layers of brick to their wall . . . but in the end, you are the Cassandra here, you "see" what they can't and what others, all of us living in this toxic cancer-causing culture, need to see.

It sounds like the ongoing raw and Dr. A's treatments are truly healing, of both spirit and body. I'm sure it feels like you're flying solo. You're already a miracle man, but I want very much for you to be a Miracle Man in this, too. You are being humble and just Living As You Must now, deeply quietly hoping I'm sure for total remission because of these self-loving treatments. Surely this self-loving is the way. We all want this for you, rescue from the trauma of all this by this brave and loving path, and a long life of Art and Companionship and a Sense of the Possible.

So thanks to you and Ann for this update, and know there is only support for your choices and your Much Improved Health in this post allopathic period. It *is* such a gift that most of your symptoms have been reduced or eliminated by the treatments you're pursuing. You are creating an environment that is increasingly inhospitable to cancer. You probably know this great quote by Mao (quoted by Zizek last week in relation to Egypt): "There is chaos under heaven—the situation is excellent!" *Exactly!*

Much love and thawing, rawing, toward spring—

BETH, WITH OF COURSE LOVE FROM PETER, TOO!

ENDING THE TERATOGENIC-CARCINOGENIC-IATROGENIC MATRIX

A good friend (who shall remain nameless) persists in trying to advocate that I do the rectal-removal surgery, even despite my repeated statements to him that I will not do this, nor will I participate anymore in the allopathic system. His argument is simple: the surgery will remove the entire area for which these so-far nonmetastasic tumors have aggressively appeared. He has not heard me continue repeating that extending my life at the cost to my dignity and my quality of living is not an acceptable trade-off anymore. Furthermore, as I reflect back upon the last four years of allopathic treatments, including multiple surgeries, and as the increasing belief even among the allopathic establishment grows, that cancer may actually be exacerbated and spread by such treatments, he still persists contrary to my wishes. There is a growing belief that repeated mammograms may actually increase risk for breast cancer. That the radiation from the CT/PT scans do the same. That surgeries actually disperse and spread cancer cells. This is the fundamental conundrum to technocentric and technocratic medicine: creating more problems while never being real solutions. The cut–burn–poison matrix of the CIME cannot be a solution because it is a paradigm that addresses effects and not causes, services the superprofits of big pharma and medical institutions preoccupied with management of illness and dependency upon these protocols and institutions, and finally, unable to supplant these institutions and protocols with a culture and system of wellness, prevention and self—and communal healing.

I have reached the conclusion early on in this war that capitalism is the cancer for the planet (eco-cide), while the exponential increase in social and environmental toxicity of capitalism is cancer for the individual person. It is this nexus that must be understood and to which solutions must be targeted. Individually, as I've come to believe, we can only chip away by struggling to extricate our existence from the matrix. Collectively, we must end the capitalist mode of production/existence, that matrix of the teratogenic, the carcinogenic and the iatrogenic.

Many of these ideas are expressed in a searingly beautiful work, "Every Time I Open My Mouth to Sing," lyrics written by the great poet Jayne Cortez and for which I composed music to be performed by baritone voice (Tom Buckner) and baritone sax (myself). We have two premieres: in San Francisco at the Herbst Theater; and at Roulette, 20 Greene Street, in Manhattan. Please come!

All love,

FRED

DIARY 31: TURNING THE CORNER, FACING THE TRUTH

March 18, 2011

For everyone who has been reading my cancer war diaries since they began in the early fall of 2006, some good days and mostly bad days has been the norm. But since beginning my alternative, naturopathic treatments, that has been reversed: now mostly good days and some bad days.

In the past four diaries, I have recounted on how profound my life has changed, and for the first time in the four-year cancer war, I truly have confidence and hope that I will be able to beat cancer.

However, recently, more bad days have been occurring that have included severe fatigue, constant rectal pain, more blood discharge from my anus, but these only occurred on days for which I was not getting my alternative treatments. On the days for which I was getting these treatments, this adverse feeling was quickly corrected; pumped with oxygen, I felt like cancer had been beaten.

After constant repeat of this up-and-down cycle, I was getting very concerned that my alternative treatments were more palliative than curative, and feeling doubts, my anxiety about dying started to grow.

Because of the sensitivity of my specific alternative treatments (for which the majority of states in the United States regard as illegal), I have in these diary pages refrained from directly discussing or revealing what my oxygen therapy has entailed. But I began to do much more research, and from all accounts, both from American and international accounts, my specific therapies are regarded very positively, not only as a treatment for cancer but also for many other maladies.

During the course of my alternative treatments since they began in early December 2010, I have been making a growing circle of friends at Dr. Bill's office. I have referred two good friends, Idel and John, to him, and they have become regulars and have enjoyed and benefited from his treatments. My cancer war diaries have been read by another patient, Gibi, who have found in them great spiritual succor and validation of her decision to forego the allopathic for the naturopathic. She and I have especially shared some humor about the institutional arrogance of Memorial Sloan-Kettering, who gave her only six months to live from a stage 4 colon-liver cancer prognosis.

Gibi had come to Dr. Bill's about two weeks prior to me, and she was a wreck (who wouldn't be if told by the celebrated doctors of MSK that they only had six months to live). I witness Dr. Bill's controversial treatments upon her and at that moment, seeing it for myself, believed that something powerful and unconventional was being done. Gibi now, after four months, radiates health and happiness. We joked about her recent visit to Dr. Saltz, her oncologist at MSK who gave her the bleak prognosis, that when she, a former model, would strut into his office, doing her runway walk and dressed to the nines, and shock him with her strength and vitality. I said to Gibi that if he asks you what you've been doing, since you decided not to listen to him, rejected his prescription and prognosis, to tell him, with a straight face, that you've been doing the Fred Ho protocol.

Well, Gibi did it! She tells me that after she told him with a straight face that that was what she had done, she reported that he quizzically asked, "What's that?" She told him the truth: chapparal tea, diet change, and oxygen therapies. He replied, "I don't know anything about that." We both laughed: Of course you don't!

My new circle of friends at Dr. Bill's office, fellow patients, have been mutually sharing experiences and information about our respective struggles, including various materials on alternative protocols. I have devised my own methods that include as a foundation Dr. Bill's treatments as well as those I've devised and added, periodically experimenting with new options, incorporating or discarding these as I try them out and see their effect or lack of effect. This has added a fifth principle to my strategy of fighting cancer: in addition to hydration, nutrition, oxygenation, and love, I now add *self-healing*. Taking charge of one's treatment and recovery, no longer passively and loyally following allopathic or any protocols, to learn to truly know one's body, to be in command of improving one's health, to make boldly make decisions even when they countermand and contravene allopathic doctors and their protocols.

So this past Saturday, feeling weak and awful, I arrived early at Dr. Bill's office and told his staff that I was not doing well. Soon after Dr.

Bill arrived, he saw me. He responded to my anxiety with the nobility of character that should be a model for all working in the health care profession. He said to me, "Fred, I will make sure you don't die. I will die for you before I let that happen to you." He made the immediate decision to increase my dosage of a particular therapy threefold. As he put it, "We're gonna nuke that tumor." He even advanced more experimental protocols for me that day. In minutes, I could feel my life force elevating, and by the time I returned home, I was reborn, renewed, and reinvigorated.

To relieve the pain in my anus, I am now applying green tea extract, soaking my butt in hydrogen peroxide bathwater with MMS and organic ozonated olive oil.

Within a couple of days, I began to feel a marked change and improvement. I believe that I've turned a corner in the cancer war and headed for victory. As I've described, I can tell from now knowing my body whether I have cancer and how it is doing. I now feel that the tumor is being nuked, hammered, pulverized, that the retreat has begun. It still is too early to tell. But an interesting development, possibly the karma in the universe working, occurred today, March 16, 2011, at 3:10 PM.

I had just gotten back to my apartment after a relaxing and enjoyable lunch at Sharaku Restaurant, my large midday meal (I don't eat any later than 7:00 PM, and my later meal is a small one) consisting of a mixed seaweed salad, six varieties of raw fish, and brown rice. The phone rang, and I picked it up. If I had caller ID, I probably would not have picked up this call, but to my surprise it was Dr. Jason Bratcher, the gastroenterologist at Beth Israel who had ignominiously cancelled my ultrasound scan back in January.

Rather than hang up or get mad, I engaged him in a vigorous conversation, saying you can hear the strength and vigor in my voice. I'm doing great (no thanks to you and the allopathic doctors). He said he had called to see how I was doing (maybe he had read my blog?). I told him I was doing a bevy of alternative, naturopathic treatments for which I couldn't discuss with him since they are "off the reservation." I could tell that there was contrition from him. I told him that I won't accept surgery again, that getting a fifth tumor after an irreversible procedure as the surgeons wanted was not acceptable to me, that I would commit suicide if that happened, and that I was determined to find a solution, that the allopathic paradigm offered no solutions, and how would he respond if I indeed found a solution, that if I could beat cancer?

He was humbled. He couldn't accept that his paradigm could be proven wrong. I said to him if would he do another ultrasound scan to prove me wrong, or to see for himself that I had found a way to beat this tumor. He extended a sincere and humble agreement to do an ultrasound scan but made the caveat that if I was wrong, was I prepared to accept suffering and death if I didn't accept the surgery protocol. I said I had already come to peace with myself: either I beat cancer naturopathically, or I die. I have seen death all around me: other cancer patients fading before me, dialysis patients (who have lost both kidneys) still alive but not really living anymore—this is what my sister Flora had questioned me: was I ready to accept death? And the answer now is without any doubt or hesitation: yes, either victory or death, and that I would commit suicide if I couldn't beat cancer.

I was surprised, but after we hung up, I was pleased that Dr. Bratcher called me, both for his genuine human caring and for my increased desire to show all of the allopathic doctors that cancer can be beaten naturopathically, and to knock down any bit of their smug certainty about their paradigm. Dr. Bratcher conceded that he couldn't dismiss the effects of diet and exercise and said he was open to seeing the results of my treatments. I said I would call him in two months for him to do this ultrasound scan that he now promised to do.

Since being diagnosed with cancer for this fourth time, I flew on an airplane to the Bay Area to perform with singer Thomas Buckner. The concert went off well, but the jet lag and physical toll of flying had hammered me for almost five days. We did the concert again a few days after San Francisco in New York City on a terribly rainy night, though with a warm and receptive full house. Don Chow was visiting, and he joined Gibi, Idel, John, and I for a great Chinese meal at Congee in Chinatown. During these concert activities, Tom has been a wonderful friend, always asking how I'm feeling and making sure my physical demands aren't too stressful. Playing my big baritone sax in the way I do is quite a workout!

I also recently learned that I will be receiving the Guggenheim Fellowship in Music Composition. I told my family and close friends as the award hasn't been officially announced at the time of this diary issuance. My friend Arthur Song, retired and now living in Cairo (wow, what a time to be there!), e-mailed me to say this:

> Fred man, you deserve it. After passing you over for more than twenty years, it's about time. Composers who've gotten that award haven't created your body of work, its uniqueness and daring, in either the jazz or classical worlds. They kept rejecting you because of your explicit radical politics as these art-for-art's sake ideologues can't conceive that you can be politically committed and engaged, outside of and against this system, and still be an artist. To them, it is not only inconceivable you are who you are, but wrong.

I jokingly replied that after such a long string of rejections, I don't need or expect the money and would blow it on a party for the Warriors for Fred and give almost all of it away! Which is what I intend to do, so look out for the party announcement after the award is announced and I get the dough.

If I had done the surgery to remove my entire rectum and have a permanent colostomy bag, I probably now would be only getting back my strength, walking again, and returning to my activity. I'm so happy that I didn't do the surgery, as many tremendous things would have been sacrificed, including the developing of several young revolutionary leaders in my collection the *Scientific Soul Sessions* (www.scientificsoulsessions.com). We are in the thick of planning this year's sessions/events and many other projects and elevating a new revolutionary praxis.

I will be continuing the cancer war diary for as long as I am fighting cancer, but should cancer not be beaten and I die, either from its ravage or by my own volition, I am happy that I have had the chance to share my graphic experiences and hard-fought lessons, which will hopefully gain a wider audience with the September publication of these diaries as a book. It is because of my May 1, 2011, deadline to finalize the book that I end this entry.

In a couple of days, I'm headed to Bocas del Toro islands in Panama to snorkel and be among the ocean life, taking a break from thinking about and fighting the cancer war. I am seriously trying to tick off my bucket list (a list of what one wants to do before kicking the bucket), including snorkeling with the biggest pelagics in the ocean!

All love,

FRED HO

MEDITATION OF SOME FINAL THOUGHTS ON THE CANCER WAR

The U.S. government and the mainstream medical establishment declared an official war on cancer in the 1970s. That war has been an abject failure. More cancers have been diagnosed. More deaths from all cancers have dramatically risen (the once-hailed "decline in breast and colon cancers" are now shown to be statistical misreadings and possible chicanery).

Why? How can a cure be touted if a cause cannot be ascribed? There is no singular cause, no genetic engineering that will fix the accelerative malignancy generated by the industrial capitalist matrix, a matrix of exponentially increasing social and environmental toxicity, severe weakening of natural and biological immune and corrective processes from this massive assault.

With the imminent meltdown of nuclear energy reactors (unfolding as I write this in Japan, and for which other disasters in many other countries will soon to follow), for which the presumption of nuclear safety is a grand oxymoron, and for which there is no possible safe containment of nuclear waste (which has a toxic life of about a quarter of a million years), cancers of all kinds will be multiplying, from both direct contamination of humans, to water and food sources, which quickly reach humans.

Dr. Bill Akpinar made the statement, "Everyone has cancer. It's just the matter of each individual's tipping point." In my personal war against cancer, I have tried to extend my tipping point, through optimizing my personal health from the raw/organic extreme diet revolution, to working on an organic farm with all of its attendant benefits (exercise, fresh mountain air, sweat therapy, nutritionally dense food, space and time to be Zen, etc.), to at first following diligently, faithfully, and loyally the allopathic protocols, to their outright rejection for the naturopathic (and devising the Fred Ho protocol, see below), to devising my five-point strategy for waging war against cancer (hydration, nutrition, oxygenation, love, and self-healing), to making my self-dignity and quality of life paramount (and extending my love, generosity, and friendship to all of the Warriors for Fred in as many ways as I can). I have killed the old Fred Ho and taken this cancer war as a gift and opportunity to make the

New Fred Ho. And I have accepted the way of the warrior: to live while preparing for death.

I have created my best music and innovated some of the most imaginative political theories for revolutionary change, embodied in the very young collection *Scientific Soul Sessions* (www.scientificsoulsessions.com). I have taken on the mission to do the impossible: what no one else can or will not do in terms of art and politics. I have eliminated personal ego, though anger still claws at me as long as I have a conscience, compassion, and caring about making a qualitatively better future.

And yet, I still have not beaten cancer. I may never win, though for the first time, I feel optimistic (and not the typical and usual feelings of anger and depression after leaving allopathic medical appointments and treatments). My days are very uneven, some fantastic days when I feel cancer is defeated, to tired and painful days of feeling like my life force is waning.

I have tried to write these diaries without the mellifluous platitudes of hope and cheerful optimism. The war against cancer has been brutal, rough, horrific, and has taken its toll upon me. In these diaries, I have pulled no punches, masked no difficulties, and explicitly revealed the ravages upon my physical and psychic being. I realized early in the war that I would have to be profoundly changed for the better, to be the New Fred Ho. Whether I live or die, that understanding and transformation was worth extending my life, but to be that New Fred Ho meant more than continuing to stay alive; it has meant defining what living must be if we are to exit this material world, the summation of our contributions and efforts.

One last commentary on the conundrum of complementary medicine (or the proposition of combining the allopathic with the alternative). While in some cases, such a mixture is effective, usually with the allopathic being primary and the alternative as secondary, and usually as a palliative supplement, in most cases, the combination is fundamentally conflictive. For example, after surgery or during chemotherapy, the allopathic prescription is for the patient to continue of a low-residue diet, which is weak nutritionally. Raw food, high-fiber foods, and nuts are all disallowed in this protocol. After one of my surgeries, I tried to follow a naturopathic diet, which resulted in awful diarrhea and suffering. In these cases, the two ways are irreconcilable. Postchemotherapy, sweat therapy is a key way to rid the body of the devastating chemo toxins.

I must stress that for every individual, what pathway you chose depends upon the severity of the cancer and the strength of yourself. There are no prescriptions. Each person must learn to know their body and soul, be constantly open to change, and trying new treatments and healing activities.

In the end, there are a few things that these conflicted paradigms agree upon to be important, perhaps key, components to either beating cancer or fighting cancer in the best possible way: the strength of the individual's spirit and diet and exercise and the overall wellness and optimizing of a person's health before, during, and following treatments.

I wish I had the understanding of what I have now, especially of avoiding high-temperature-cooked foods, of the importance of raw extremism, and a pro-Luddite orientation, including a far greater respect for the naturopathic.

That is why I have written these diaries, why they are presented in real-time, to show the journey and development, the twists and turns, the mistakes, the failings, the transformations, and the lessons.

I have vowed that a fifth tumor is unacceptable. I will commit suicide. It will mean that solutions, for myself at least, are not possible, that my making a tipping point in which my treatments and transformations will be sufficient to keep cancer cells at bay will never be attained. That my case, while not hopeless, was essentially too late and beyond making a new tipping point to have at least attained a lifespan of an added ten years from diagnosis.

Only time will tell, along with huge spirit and ongoing struggle for solutions.

Endnotes

1. I have excerpted Jay's e-mail dated August 9, 2007 below:

    "For some years now I have believed that cancer and capitalism are really the same process, simply in two different forms. Process is the essential reality of all things. Heraclitus said that 2,500 years ago, and Whitehead told us again in a somewhat more obscure manner. And the process that is cancer and is capitalism is, of course, uncontrolled growth. Uncontrolled growth at the cellular level is cancer and at the socioeconomic level is capitalism. Same process, different form. And just as uncontrolled growth at the cellular level destroys the physical body, so uncontrolled growth at the social level destroys the social body. It does not take a genius to see this, but the myths and propaganda issuing from the ruling class hide from the masses the cancerous nature of the consumer culture that they willingly participate in. This makes it much more difficult to fight capitalism effectively than it is to fight cancer. Cancer is openly fatal. Capitalism is secretly fatal. A raging ignorance stalks the land, Fred and I fear that ignorance will successfully conceal the destructiveness of capitalism until it reeks havoc and death (of course, it already is, but I mean on a massive scale in a short amount of time) across the planet. I wish I could be more optimistic, but I see nothing in man's history to enable that optimism."

2. My sister Florence has rethought this growth time and more recently hypothesizes that the tumor took less time to grow to such enormity given that the particular colorectal cancer cells found within me might be more intensely accelerative since the recurrence came back so quickly, so aggressively, and of considerable growth.

3. In fall of 2007, the oncologist Dr. Peter Kozuch told me he thought I had about one in four chances of living. Recurrence with such accelerated and aggressive characteristics as in the case of my cancer war did not leave much basis for optimism. Former White Press press secretary for President George W. Bush, Peter Snow, originally staged at 2b colorectal cancer (lower than my stage 3b) did not survive the recurrence. Of course, he did not have the warriors I had and continued to commit his life and soul to the perpetuation of great evil, namely U.S. imperialism, with fervidness that furthered his immersion into profound levels of toxicity.

PREFIGURATIVE PRELUDE: AN AFTERWORD

This cancer war diary from 2006 to mid-2011 has no conclusion. I wish I could say that I've beaten cancer, but I haven't. An often-quipped saying "What is more important are the questions asked then the answers" is very apt to my struggle.

My personal war against cancer has raised many questions, which have become contentions against everything conventionally understood, espoused, prescribed, contemplated, and conveyed about cancer in America, and how to fight it.

The mainstream medical establishment's so-called war on cancer began in the 1970s has clearly been an abject failure, as more and more types of cancers are being diagnosed and rates are alarmingly increasing, especially in the affluent societies such as ours, and deaths are also increasing for almost all types of cancer, though early detection for certain types (primarily colorectal, which is what I've faced, and breast cancer) has meant better success rates at curative treatments.

My alternative, naturopathic doctor said this to me: "Everyone has cancer. It's just a matter of each person's particular tipping point." He also made no promises he could cure me, saying that "Fred, we're going for a miracle, but miracles have been known to happen!" Miracles are not within the purview of the mainstream cancer industrial complex. Too often, in metastatic cases, or for which repeated recurrences have manifested, allopaths tell their patients, "You only have X number of months or at the most X number of years to live." Clearly, for myself, with repeated recurrences, I have beaten the odds and predictions. But I am not cured and perhaps may never be cured. What I have been able to do is to move the tipping point (though not to the ten-year mark that I was hoping for, at least not yet) by optimizing my mind-body-spirit connection, to become a Zen warrior in the war against cancer.

Early on in the cancer war, I recognized the matrix between cancer and capitalism, as being the same accelerative malignant processes (not just a disease, but an exponential increasing interaction between teratogenic-carcinogenic acceleration, which given the at best, myopia and, at worst, refusal, to understand and address this matrix, has resulted in the addition of the iatrogenic (death caused by allopathic institutions and practitioners and specifically by the mainstream cancer industrial complex). It is my contention that a technocentric cure is impossible for cancer. Only a reversal of the saturated social and environmental toxicity (from physical to consumerist obesity, waste, pollution, and eco-cide) will a cure become possible. The biggest deception is to even contend that a cure can be found when the causes aren't either known or are misguidedly sought in biotechnical engineering (the genetics causation argument).

While humans have had cancer for a long time, indeed the span of most of civilization, as carcinogens have been present (such as smoke and eating burnt food), it is with the rise of the cancerlike spread of industrialism has cancer become pervasive across the globe and inevitably present in every human society.

My journey in the cancer war, which is a global and epic war, both against an exponentially expanding malignant matrix, has two parts, and I would say, two kinds of wars. From 2006–2010, I was the perfect cancer patient, spurning and dismissive of the naturopathic or alternative modalities, and completely committed and loyal to the allopathic. However, by the end of 2010, after being under the cancer of the supposedly best cancer institution in the United States, and perhaps the world, Memorial Sloan-Kettering, it became evident that no solutions were going to be found in this paradigm, only more of the same treatments with potentially greater and more severe losses to my quality of life and physical and spiritual being. And after costs that well exceeded $1 million, as I began to have the smallest curiosity about nonallopathic therapies, the institutional arrogance of the allopathic practitioners, I quickly came to see that their paradigm was about cancer management (which is infinitely more profitable) than effecting solutions, especially since solutions may very well be nonpharmaceutical and not require the considerable billable expenditures of large institutions. My rejection of allopathy was quick and decisive, and I have become a pariah to those institutions and everyone ideologically and financially tethered to them.

In the first part of my cancer war, I self-devised a basic strategy to fighting cancer: *oxygenation, hydration, nutrition, and love.* The naturopathic path continues with this strategy, but since I am no longer shackled to industrial medicine, the creative and practical possibilities for these four components has dramatically broadened and deepened.

I completely reject the notion of complementary medicine. In such a formulation, mainstream medicine continues to be primary, and the naturopathic is subordinate. Neither allopathic or alternative medicine, as long as the capitalist matrix dominates either, can present solutions, only more profiteering that promulgates the acquisitive. Wellness and health and cures are diametrically opposed to profiteering. Health and quality of life must never be compromised or corrupted by money, stratified and dominated by either those who have or enjoy it (from wealthier patients to the institutions and their underlings who are employed toward the furtherance of accumulating wealth for capitalist medicine), or those who lack it and are denied or excluded from quality care.

Since my paradigm shift, I would add a fifth component to my strategy: *self-healing*, combining autodidactic and collaborative approaches. This is the taboo subject, the forbidden zone, for mainstream doctors whose elevated stature in society ("Marry a doctor or a lawyer!") would quickly be dethroned if the doctor-patient relation was eliminated, or even if patients realized the problem of iatrogenic harm and refused on faith or timidity to not concede to everything that they are instructed to do. By sharing experiences and experimental treatment information, the patients in Dr. Akpinar's office became a support group and healing society. This is the prefiguration to a potentially better system of medicine in which people are put first and not paradigms, protocols, or profits. Albeit short of destroying the industrial capitalism economic-social-cultural-psychological-medical matrix, we cancer fighters, along with wellness practitioners, are working to change our personal lives and practices, to maximize our natural immune systems as the principal method in fighting cancer (and other maladies), to better our individual spirits and turn the fear and brutality of cancer into liberating flowers and gardens of a better humanity for which each individual person is that seed and progenitor.

Live or die, my quality of life, my spiritual being, my creative essence, my life force are stronger than ever; my philosophical visioning, my imagination and ability to sense and visualize a new and better life for myself and for humanity—all these have changed me in profound ways as I killed off the old Fred Ho and created the New Fred Ho.

When people who are told of their cancer diagnosis ask me what advice I can give to them, I say, you can take cancer as a curse, and it is horrific (and greatly made more horrible by the cut-burn-poison paradigm of mainstream medicine), or you can take it as gift, an opportunity to change yourself *forever*, to never go back to the carcinogenic matrix of the life you once lived, and to build a new person and new life that is truly better!

All love,

FRED HO (STILL ALIVE, STILL FIGHTING AS OF MAY 1, 2011)

Appendix

POSSIBLE ANTICOLORECTAL CANCER WEAPONS: THE FRED HO PROTOCOL

I have not elaborated on the possibilities listed below, as they are my own personal experimental therapies. One of my lessons is that we must find what works for each of us individually as we are all different. I am not advising anyone to initially reject allopathic treatments, only that when it feels to you that it is not working for you, to search beyond that paradigm toward the naturopathic.

The Fred Ho protocol includes the following, though not necessarily in the order of priority as presented below (please note that a number of these therapies are highly controversial, some maligned and dismissed by the allopathic paradigm, and one, ozone, illegal in thirty-seven states of the United States):

1. Selenium
2. Chinese Herbs such as shark cartilage
3. Chaparral
4. Oxygen and Ozone Therapies
5. Sweat therapy
6. Hyperbaric chamber
7. Serapin and mushroom serum extracts
8. Indole 3-carbinole

9. MMS
10. Acupuncture
11. Raw food
12. Water
13. Vitamins D and E
14. Green tea extract orally and rectally

Recommended Resources

Healers

Trina Shore Sims is a master herbalist with over forty years experience in the effective use of beneficial plants. Her company, GreenStar Herbs LLC, specializes in custom formulation for health professionals and private clients.
Website: www.greenstarherbs.com
E-mail: focus@greenstarherbs.com

Dr. Bluten (Bill) Akpinar (only open Tuesdays, Thursdays, and Saturdays from 10:00 AM to 7:00 PM), 61-10 Marathon Parkway, Douglaston, NY 11362

Charlene Muhammad, MS, Clinical Herbalist and Nutrition Consultant, www.urbanherblist.org

Books

Altman, Nathaniel. *The Oxygen Prescription: The Miracle of Oxidative Therapies.* Rochester, VT: Healing Arts Press, 2007.

Campbell, T. Colin and Campbell, Thomas M. *The China Study: The Most Comprehensive Study of Nutrition Ever Conducted and the Startling Implications for Diet, Weight Loss and Long-Term Health.* Dallas, TX: BenBella Books, 2006.

Sourcing

GardenofEveFarm.com and many other organic farms with CSAs (community-supported agriculture programs)

EatGreenpoint.com (in New York City, the most exemplary all-organic, all-local, all-vegan prix-fixe restaurant that should be the model for many more across the United States and the world!)

MountainRoseHerbs.com (all organic herbs)